To my four granddaughters,

Cienna,

Bailee,

Sailor,

and

Evie,

*for all the joy and love
you bring to my heart.*

A Guide to Energetically
Awaken You to the Pleiadian Prophecies for
Healing and Resurrection

PLEIADIAN
INITIATIONS OF LIGHT

CHRISTINE DAY

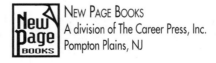
NEW PAGE BOOKS
A division of The Career Press, Inc.
Pompton Plains, NJ

PLEIADIAN INITIATIONS OF LIGHT
EDITED BY JODI BRANDON
TYPESET BY EILEEN MUNSON
Cover design by Lucia Rossman/DigiDog Design
Printed in the U.S.A.
Images created by Lisa Glynn.

To order this title, please call toll-free 1-800-CAREER-1 (NJ and Canada: 201-848-0310) to order using VISA or MasterCard, or for further information on books from Career Press.

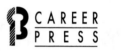

The Career Press, Inc., 220 West Parkway, Unit 12
Pompton Plains, NJ 07444
www.careerpress.com
www.newpagebooks.com

Library of Congress Cataloging-in-Publication Data

Day, Christine, 1955–
    Pleiadian initiations of light : a guide to energetically awaken you to the pleiadian prophecies for healing and resurrection / by Christine Day.
        p. cm.
    Includes index.
    ISBN 978-1-60163-099-5
    ISBN 978-1-60163-738-3
        1. Spirituality--Miscellanea. 2. Pleiades--Miscellanea. 3. Healing--Miscellanea. I. Title.

    BF1999.D39 2010
    299'.93--dc22

                                                            2009050336

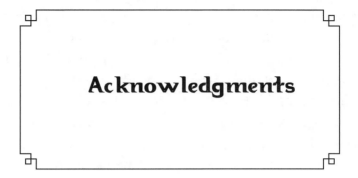

Acknowledgments

I want to start by expressing my deep appreciation for the guidance, support, and friendship of my agent, Laurie Harper, who believed in this book from the first reading, for her expertise, honesty, and dedication to the vision of this book with the CDs attached (now available as audio files at *www.christinedayonline.com/piol*). Thank you to Briah Anson for bringing my book to Laurie's attention in the first place.

To years of friendship and our deep connection, I send my love and thanks to Michael Bradley for the recording and editing of the audio tracks, for all the recordings over the years, and for your dedication and commitment to me and this work.

My love and gratitude to Lynne Bradley, for our friendship, and all the love and support you have given me.

I want to acknowledge my truly amazing daughter, Lisa Glynn, for her incredible love and support throughout the years, and for the work she has done with the diagrams and drawings for this book. My utmost love and respect for you and your journey my darling girl.

A special thank you to Efren Solanas, for your friendship, love, and encouragement through the years.

To my dearest and most treasured friends, Jo Bray, Lorelee Wederstrom, Ruth Palmer, and Susan Arthur, for being part of my family and for your support, love, and help along the way.

My many thanks to the Frequencies of Brilliance practitioners, teachers, and all my students who have held me with so much love and support throughout this journey of writing a book.

And I end with my heartfelt thanks to the love of my life, Alisa, who has been by my side through this whole process, and without her incredible support this book would not have been possible. For your presence in my life and in my heart, and for holding an energy that enables us to live "heaven on earth" while on this planet together.

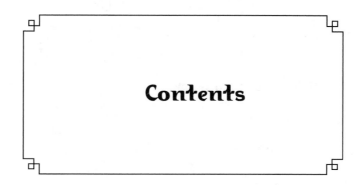

Contents

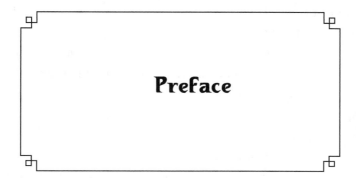

Preface

*Greetings. It is with great love that I
present this book to you.*

Over the last 22 years I have been on a journey with the
Pleiadians, coming from a place of dark despair to a place of
physical and emotional healing; to a place of understanding
and knowledge of my life mission, and a profound connection to the
light of my Self. The initiations from the Pleiadians (pronounced "plea-
aid´-ee-ans") have made this transformation possible. Without them I
would never have been able to take the steps necessary to survive and
thrive to adulthood, and come to this place of incredible transformation.

Through this deep initiation to myself I was able to open up to
the healing connections with Jesus and Mother Mary, and many other
masters and light beings. It is also through them that my transformation
continues on a daily basis.

This book holds the initiations to allow you a similar transformation.
It will not be identical to mine because each one of us is unique, and each

one of us has a unique journey back to Self. The Pleiadians have asked me to bring these initiations to you so that you, too, can transform into your own light. It is designed to assist you in aligning more completely to your energies and to awaken to your Self, so that you will be able to play your part in the anchoring of light onto the planet. There are many changes coming onto our earth plane. Our planet is going through huge dimensional changes, moving from a third-dimensional planet to a fourth/fifth-dimensional planet.

Let me explain what this means when I say that our planet is in a *third-dimensional consciousness at this time*. Throughout our planet there is a strong societal belief in our limitation and deficiency—that we are *lacking*. There is profound *fear*, which creates a mighty struggle and tiredness that permeates societies. If you are like most people, you are not in touch with your abilities—your natural and unlimited ability to create—and you do not understand the divine aspect of Self. You have the illusion of being *alone and separate,* and are unaware of the beauty and magnificence of your individual uniqueness within the Universe. And over most of the planet, *time* is probably one of the biggest illusions; that time exists. *The belief in time* creates incredible limitation to reality. So this is a brief outline of the third-dimensional consciousness, to which I refer.

Fourth-dimensional consciousness means being part of something greater than ourselves. None of us are alone. You begin to be aware of the spiritual energies around you and are able to open up to the support that is here for you. Fear begins to drop away and does not control your experience. There is a connection to your heart, and intuitive guidance coming to you from an aspect of the Self through this connection to the heart. Your Sacred heart begins to work with you in your day-to-day life, awakening you to the true life force that moves through all living beings and all living matter. You begin to understand and experience your place within the universal consciousness and begin to move with the intuitive guidance of the Self. There is a strong sense of purpose, and you begin to feel passionate about life. There is a sense of freedom and deep experience of love, and you begin to be fed by that love, opening up to all living beings.

Fifth-dimensional consciousness is moving into a state of unconditional love—a state of oneness with all life consciousness, having a direct experience of being one with the Universal consciousness, and having a conscious steady alignment to the pure love of your God essence. You remember your place within this universal consciousness and begin linking into your unlimited potential to create. You awaken to your natural gifts of creativity, remembering your full birthright to be able to manifest abundance on all levels for yourself, taking back your power of full manifestation. You remember your mission here on this earth plane. There is no fear—only an experience of love.

Moving from a third-dimensional state of consciousness to a fourth/fifth-dimensional state is exciting and powerful for all of us, and you have an important role to play in this transformation. If you have not experienced being part of the universal consciousness—of being part of the oneness—this book is designed to open you into this awareness and a direct connection to the Self. It is also designed to deepen your alignment and take you into new levels of initiation with yourself that will align you more completely with direct experiences and deeper connections to your God Self. You have only to trust and follow your guidance. The chapters take you through a step-by-step process. The Pleiadians will hold energetic platforms for you to initiate into, which will bring you to an alignment with the light of your Self.

You might ask, "What are platforms?" Platforms are like energetic holograms: pure in form and complete in themselves. An energetic platform is held for each one of you as you work through this book. Like a mirror, it is held up so that you can move into and align to the full form of the Self. It is held steady so that you can move and match the vibration of yourself, flowing into your own initiation. This is the commitment of the Pleiadians: to hold each one of you that gives your permission for this help. It will not be activated unless you give your permission. The Pleiadians honor each one of us, and our right to choose. We are allowed to say yes one moment and no the next, so you can change your mind at any time.

As you move and initiate into this awakening, you begin to take your place more completely in life. With the birth of the Self you are able to move into the work that you have come here to do at this time on this planet.

Becoming more awakened brings us into a different state of consciousness. We actually have a different vibration in our cells. It's a frequency of love, and it naturally flows as we move through the world. It affects the people around us, and all living things.

Some people are afraid to allow these changes to take place, because they don't know what these changes are going to bring to them in their lives. How are things going to change? It's important to understand that your free will is in tact and you will not have to do anything that does not feel right for you. It may be that you will just live, and transmit that vibration of love through the planet wherever you go. That is enough; you are enough!

Many of us here on the earth plane will be playing roles in holding energetic spaces and alignments during this time, in order for this transformation of the earth plane to take place. There is going to be a resurrection of our planet—a new level of love anchored here on this earth plane. This change is going to open up the hearts of people, activating a self-realization process and bringing everyone into new connections to the universal consciousness and to their own divine aspect of the oneness. Because of these coming changes it is important for you to be more conscious in the part that you are playing here now and become aware of the connections to your Self. It is important that you become more consciously connected to the Spiritual energies that are here to assist you, as you align more and more to your own light. This conscious connection that I speak about is important because you choose the moments to align; you choose the moment to take each step.

When I talk about Spiritual energies I refer to the Light beings: the Angels and the Masters of Light that are here with us. They are committed to helping with our unfolding and opening. And of course you have the Pleiadians at your side to help you.

The Pleiadians have asked me to write this book to assist you in finding your way back to your Self—to resurrect your Self in alignment to your light—so that you too can be your own healer and conduit on this earth plane. As your awareness of the Pleiadians presence, the Spiritual realms, and the Natural forces grow you will be able to utilize all the gifts and support that are here for you in the journey of your birth. The Pleiadians hold an unconditional loving space for you as you move toward this transition, assisting each of us who asks for their help. When called, they are committed to assisting you as you realign to a remembrance of who you really are in your unlimited state of Self.

When you open up to your Self you will become able to play your part more fully and consciously in this transition of the earth, because you will have a greater awareness of the energies around you. The planet needs more people living in this consciously connected state with Spirit, awakening to the light of themselves, and consciously anchoring their light onto the planet. As you take your place, you can then play an active part in helping to anchor all light energies on the planet. As you participate in this way you will be accelerating your own self-realization process, expanding your Sacred heart, deepening your connection to the Self. One action feeds the other, building your essence of love and connection to your place within the Universal consciousness.

You have been waiting and wanting to feel deeply satisfied within and to align more and more to the Self. Deep inside you have known that you are here to do something important, though you have not known what that is. In this moment you do not need to know the details or the steps you need to take to move toward this role. All you need to do is to take a breath and open to the processes in this book. Each process will take you on a journey, and each journey will bring you into more clarity. It will happen. Step by step, moment by moment, breath by breath.

I will be with you as you move through each step of this initiation of your light. You will not be alone in this journey. You will be united with others on a similar path and together you will align. There are many who will be called, and many who are already awakened and opening up to their mission and the work they have come here to do.

You have chosen to be here on the earth plane at this time. It is a great privilege that you are here now. Your unique energies are needed to support the planet before, during, and after the transition. I know it is hard for you to imagine or to see yourself this way, but *you are unique. There is only one of you.* Your unique energy is important, and you are needed at this time. It is time for you to align with the people like yourself and to form communities and work together, supporting each other in your transitions of your light Selves. In doing this you support the energy here on the planet.

It is important to become part of a community, which can be two or more people who are committed to their journeys of awakening: people who are willing to witness the birth in each other, allowing each person to be all he or she needs to be in each moment, and to witness the letting go of the old structures of Self and supporting the birth of the new awakened Self.

As you move into a deeper level of awakening you will connect with many other people who are here to support you, whom you, in turn, will support. This is how *soul families* come together, joining in mutual awakenings.

You are ready for this: There is nothing you have to wait for. It is your time now.

We celebrate all that you are. There is no other person like you within the Universal Whole, and your uniqueness is required to complete the whole. Like a jigsaw puzzle, you hold a unique piece for a completion to take place within the scheme of things within this spiritual evolution that is unfolding on the planet, and you are needed in your fullest form. You have been given a grace period to move and unfold yourself into the initiation of your own light. There has never been such opportunity to align with the Self so quickly as now.

Who are you? What are you? What are you doing here on this earth plane at this time? What is the purpose of your journey here? You will find your answers as you move through the processes of this book. You can open to a direct experience of communication with the Pleiadians (if you choose) and the Spiritual realms. It contains a series of initiations that will begin to align you with the Self, opening you up to receive the knowledge and the truth of the steps you need to take on your journey. You will begin to be able to source the answers from the Self, in a step-by-step process. You will be able to take back your power in this lifetime and be a co-creator of your world. This is your *divine right.*

You have to be open to allowing yourself to receive. Otherwise you will continually sabotage yourself by not allowing yourself to receive the abundance and healing that are part of your natural birthright. You are going to have to allow your heart, to consciously say *yes,* to allow the openings, then walk through the doors that open. Don't hesitate; just trust and breathe and let go. Walk through the opened doors!

In the beginning the mind will not cooperate with these changes, so you are going to have to feel the fear and do it anyway.

The natural instinct for human beings when feeling fear is to contract, to close themselves off from their senses, to close down the feeling, and to freeze. The best way to conquer fear is to consciously move toward the feeling and breath. Be conscious of feeling the fear as you move forward. As you do this, the fear dissolves. Fear is just a feeling; it cannot hurt you. Don't be afraid of your feelings. Feel and continue to move forward.

You are the only one who can stop yourself from achieving these goals. You have unlimited help and *you are not alone.* The spiritual help is with you, and the Pleiadians support you if you give them the permission to do so. When you begin to open up and ask for assistance it will be there. As Spirit often asked me at times during my journey: "Why have a grain of sand when you can have the whole beach?" It is your divine right to be abundant! They ask you to be specific in what it is you need; the more specific you are in the details of what you need, the better. Then it can be created exactly the way that you need it to be.

Throughout the book we will be doing exercises to open up barriers in the heart so that you can receive from the universe, and receive aspects of your own light—aspects of your Self. When I talk about "the light of the Self" I mean the higher light aspect of you. This will help you to evolve and awaken to your true path. You connect and align with this loving, light aspect of your Self through your heart. As you align more with your heart in the initiations, you will begin to align with the true heart energy of love, and it is this love that activates the self-healing process. Your heart will go through its own transformation as you do this and will birth itself into the energy of the Sacred heart.

The truth is that you are your own healer, and only you can align with that loving, light aspect of your Self. No one else can do it for you. You will begin to open and connect yourself to the love that is present throughout the universe: the unconditional love of the Universal Consciousness. You are a part of this.

There are wounds that you carry within your heart that need to be healed. Some of these wounds have been with you for lifetimes. It is time for you to heal so that you can move forward in your life. The open wounds keep you separated from the love that is your natural birthright to experience in this lifetime. The opening of your heart with this new aspect of love will create a healing and new sense of well-being within you; it will create a new sense of Self as you feel and experience yourself differently—not apart and separate but *connected,* a part of something very beautiful and whole.

I work directly with the Pleiadians and the Spiritual realms, holding this platform for people to make the journey back to the Self. I work with many aspects of my multi-dimensional self, which makes it possible for me to work with many people at the same time effortlessly. This comes from my unlimited source of energy, so it does not deplete me in any way. Know that I am able to hold this platform for you also as you take this journey.

Be patient with yourself as you take this journey. There is a track on the website (*www.christinedayonline.com/piol/*) for each chapter that will increasingly align you, each moment, to the *Self.* The tracks will align you with the Spiritual forces, the Pleiadians, and the Natural forces. These alignments will help you to unfold into your Self, and accelerate you into a new awareness of life and truth.

Each track has an unlimited potential in its ability to assist you as you transform and birth into your energies. As you expand you will be able to utilize and work with the more expanded energetics that are held and transmitted within the audio files. Each time you listen to the same audio file it will appear very different from the previous journey that you have taken. There is an unlimited amount that you can source from, and connect into within each journey.

Know how deeply loved and held you are as you move forward to meet and celebrate yourself! You will remember and understand the truth. So be it!

With love and blessings,
Christine Day

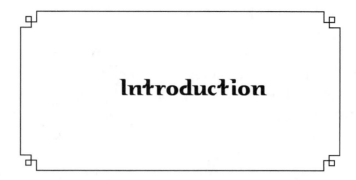

Introduction

Many of us feel that something is missing from life, and indeed it is. What's missing is our connection to the Universal Consciousness, the love aspect of the union of belonging to all living things that hold this consciousness. You are an important part of this. Without you and the gift of all that you are, the universe is incomplete. Even though this is something difficult for the ego mind to grasp, your heart understands the truth of it.

It is time for you to begin to celebrate your uniqueness and to do so consciously through your heart and out into the world. Celebrate yourself as the gift to the world.

As you move through each initiation you will begin to glimpse your new relationship to Spirit and to your Self. There is a part of your heart muscle that will begin to link you into the universal heartbeat as your heart begins to transform. Your life will begin to align with this pulse; your cells will begin to vibrate differently, and there will be a new sense of vitality taking place within your body from this connection. With this new vibration you will automatically begin to align more fully with all life, experiencing a sense of oneness with all things. Your life will transform as your vibration changes. You will draw to you new experiences of abundance, taking your power back and opening into your natural birthright of abundance on all levels.

You are not alone with your questions; you are not alone in your pain; and you are not alone in your experiences. We all have our stories, and through our stories we have an opportunity to birth ourselves back to wholeness. Your story can help you take initial steps in your journey, but there comes a time when you have to let go of your story. You cannot move into a true healing until you are willing to let go of your story. It allows you to move to a new level of healing, away from being the victim, and to take responsibility for the part you played to have your experience. This allows us to come fully back to ourselves so true healing can take place. There comes a moment when the story we have lived can no longer help us move forward. You have learned all that you can from it. You will understand that you don't have to hold on to it anymore. You don't have to hold on to the pain, the grief, the guilt, the anger, or the burdens that belong to that story. It is as though the story has become an empty shell that you no longer need to carry around with you. It is what you have identified with up to this moment, but now you know that you are much, much more than your story. In that moment of awakening you take a huge leap forward toward the Self.

It can be a scary and exciting moment when you come to this truth, and it takes great courage to let go of the story and move forward toward the Self, into a new life and a new way of living. Through these initiations you will be able to begin to move through the pain and open to the truth of the moment, the truth of the Self in this moment, and to be able to let go. Let go of the limited third-dimensional story that you have believed yourself to be, that limited you, and that held you in a cycle of self-sabotage.

We have all clung to a concept of ourselves for so long, but freedom lies beyond this illusion. True freedom lies within, so open to the passion that lies within you—the passion that can heal you and free you from your past. The self-healing process is love, patience, and compassion for ourselves. This is powerful self-healing.

I have been greatly privileged in my birthing process to be assisted by Jesus. He has come to me many times as a great teacher and dear friend. In one of my very first experiences with Him He asked me: "When are you going to take yourself off the cross? You have come here to resurrect yourself. No one else can do this for you." I realized in that moment that I had condemned myself for so many things that I had done in my life, and my guilt was overwhelming. I had been persecuting myself over and over again. With the love and teachings of Jesus, and the understanding of what love is, I was able to forgive myself and heal. Jesus showed me that I am the only one who can resurrect myself and take myself off the cross. I had put myself on the cross and I had to take myself off. I resurrected myself slowly on many different levels, step by step. It is a journey that is deep and worthwhile, and I continue this journey today, always reminding myself that the journey is the important thing, not the destination. Jesus is my ongoing teacher, assisting me to open up to more compassion, love, and patience with myself. This unfolding energy of love is now part of the platform that I hold for many people in the world. I hold this energy for each one of you as you go through these initiations.

You deserve to be loved and to love.

You cannot expect anyone to love you until you are willing to open up to self-love and compassion for yourself.

You deserve to be abundant.

The most important thing for all human beings to understand is that it is impossible for us to be perfect. We are going to make mistakes as we move through life. We sabotage ourselves when we set ourselves up to be perfect. As human beings we are "perfectly imperfect." It is through our mistakes that we learn. It is the intention behind the action that is truly important. It is with this intention and your open heart that you can move forward and live consciously. Hold yourself with compassion and patience for the mistakes that you make, and forgive yourself as you move through your day.

When you make the commitment to begin the journey back toward the Self, it enables you to also assist others as they make their own journeys. It's what I call the "Divine Economy" of the universe. It has been set up this way so that each one of us can fully utilize the energy that is changing here on this third-dimensional planet. This energy transforms as individuals begin to take back their power, connect to their light, and open to the unlimited abundance and creativity that each one of us has.

These changes create a huge wave of light energy that begins to break down the illusions here on our planet: the illusions of a lack of abundance, struggle, and fear. As the illusions of the third dimension begin to break down, the journey back to the Self begins to accelerate for each individual. It's as though the world can utilize this energy that we have created for transformation in core issues, breaking the molds that have been perpetuated on this earth plane for lifetimes. Each time we decide to do it differently, and not let the fear of the ego stop us from moving forward, we help others move through the illusion of fear because that mold of fear breaks down. It opens a stronger potential for breaking into a new freedom and a new way of living.

How do you begin the journey of self-healing, living consciously in this way?

First, you must want to consciously change and be willing to participate in the changes within yourself. You open up to an intention to live in a conscious way, which means not allowing yourself to stay complacent. You must not settle for mediocrity but move with deliberate consciousness toward your passion, your aliveness, and your own blueprint for this lifetime.

You must be open, with a conscious awareness of the light beings and those of the angelic realms that are here to assist you. Because you have free will, you must open up and *say yes* to these connections. You must invite Spirit to be with you; invite the help of this realm to come forward to assist you now.

The Pleiadians and those in the Spiritual realms have guided me step-by-step during the last 22 years. I can trust each experience that comes to me and meet whatever that experience may be in a whole new way of consciousness. This understanding has come through a series of profound experiences and initiations from the Pleiadians and the different Spiritual forces, which have led me to connecting to aspects of my own light Self. This has aligned me with a Universal truth, and led me to a deep understanding of my journey on this earth plane in this lifetime and a deep appreciation of the many difficult experiences that I have chosen to experience here in this world since birth.

My personal experience working with the Pleiadians is that they always totally respect your personal space and never come in uninvited. This is their commitment because this is your journey. They come as teachers, opening up before you knowledge and truth assisting you to take your steps, as you are ready to move forward. They will mirror your commitment to yourself; as you show up they show up, and in each moment they hold a continual space for you to birth yourself. Their love is unwavering, and their presence is steady and true.

Without their love and constant presence in my life I would not have been able to navigate myself into this healing journey that I have experienced, bringing myself from a dark despairing place to being fulfilled and healed in my life.

Know that you are not alone;

Know that you are an important aspect of the divine whole;

Know that your light is essential within this universe;

Know that you are greatly loved and are always held within the light.

There are so many people awakening at this time, and together you will form strong *soul groups*. These soul groups or soul families who are being formed are groups of people who have made pre-agreements to come together at this time, to work together energetically, to support each other in personal transformations, and to witness each other's birth of themselves. You will find each other and be strongly connected in your journeys. This is predestined. I will hold a platform of support for all of you who choose to move with the energies of this book.

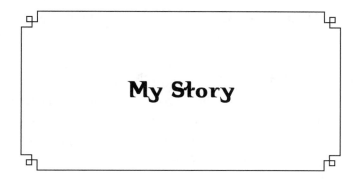

My Story

It feels important for me to share some of my life experiences with you, and the important turning points that took place at different times on my journey. We all have these turning points. I have had many.

Even though it is extremely difficult for me to go back and remember my childhood, with its loneliness, pain, and struggle, it feels important to share it with you in this book. If my experience can help any one of you, then it is worth sharing. I hope my journey inspires you when you need it. I trust the guidance of Spirit in this and I will always be deeply grateful for all that I have been through—for each experience, no matter how painful. I never want to go back and re-live any of it, but it has brought me to who I am in this moment, and to the deep, wonderful connection to my divine aspect, to a conscious recollection of all that I am, and to an understanding of my place within the Universal Consciousness.

Let me begin my story at a point in my life when I had been diagnosed with systemic lupus and been given just a few months to live.

I was 31 years old. When I heard the diagnosis, I was not so much shocked as relieved. I realized that deep inside myself I wanted to die; I had wanted to die for a long, long time.

My next thought was—and I know now looking back in retrospect, that it was an inspired thought—that I had actually created something to kill myself! I felt an excitement run through me from that realization. I hadn't believed I was capable of creating anything.

My life had been a dead life up to that point. I used to watch the clock and work out how many hours I had left in the day to live. I didn't believe I was capable of achieving anything, and had no original or creative thoughts of my own. That is why I was so excited by the thought that I was able to create this disease!

My next thought was also an inspired thought: "If I created something to kill myself, then I can also create something to heal myself!" At that moment I realized that all the pain, and all the trauma, of my childhood was somehow still locked inside of me, and I had to find a way of letting it out. I needed to find help.

I knew if I was going to live, I was going to have to find a way to do everything differently. I didn't know what that meant, but I left the hospital that day, leaving behind doctors and medicines. In retrospect, I now know that was the day I took my power back. When I walked away from the doctors and the expectation that they would heal me, I moved back toward myself knowing that I had to do something to heal me. I was responsible for my own healing! That was my healing. I didn't know it at the time—all I knew was that things had to be done differently. I wasn't sure where to begin. I wasn't connected to any church or spiritual path. I just had myself. I did know of my past, and the inspirational understanding of the pain that I still had inside of me. So I began at that place and began therapy. I had bodywork, and began a nutritional program of natural herbs. And I decided to begin to meditate daily. I had no idea how to meditate, so I just sat quietly with myself. They were the steps that I blindly chose, and they worked!

My health turned around very quickly, but then I began to deal with the deep pain of my childhood. It was crippling me emotionally and I found it very hard to navigate my way through the intense pain and fear. I was transported back to a very dark place: the place of my childhood. My memories were almost non-existent, but the feelings of emotional pain were strong and drowning me in my life. I realized that I didn't have any sense of who I was in the world, as though I had been always playing a role, almost copying other people and the way they were, rather than knowing and feeling my Self. It was a difficult time as I struggled to find myself.

I didn't really know what meditation was, but I committed to just sit still and be with myself. Gradually I became aware of some sort of peaceful presence around me, and instinctively that felt right inside of me. I had to trust the feeling; that's all I had. So I struggled with not really understanding at the time what I was doing.

One day while meditating I began receiving this amazing energy, and in a two- to three-second period two complete healing processes were given to me. It was as though I had studied the processes all of my life, and I knew them intimately.

I was overwhelmed with this experience, not knowing or trusting what was now inside of me—not only inside of me, but a part of me, not separate. It was as though a whole new part of me had been born in those two to three seconds. I sat stunned for some time, feeling me and this new part of me. I would describe it as energy and love, and something good, wholesome, and very, very real. I could feel it pulsating through my cells gently like a new heartbeat, and a light flow like a sunrise in every cell. I sat very still breathing softly and just being with this light flow. There was a definite aliveness there—aliveness I had not ever experienced in my lifetime up to that moment. Every cell was receiving a transformation and the love flowed into me, healing my cells. The love held me in a way I had never been held.

I had my son at home who had many complex health problems. A few days after receiving this energy I decided to put my hands on his body and try this work on him. As I put my hands on his body I could feel this new energy running through me. I could feel the love opening up within me and a deep sense of healing beginning to take place for me as I did the work on him. With all my doubts of my ability to be able to do this, a certain process flowed. It was easy and beautiful. It created an incredible sense of quiet joy within me. I was at peace. I was moved into a unique place of being part of something—of actually belonging somewhere for the first time in my life. And yet I could not tell you where this place existed and who I was in that place. It didn't seem to matter. Hours after working with my son I could see the changes in him. It was a miracle! It was a miracle for me and for my son.

Every day I worked with him, and every day there were healings for both of us. For two years I worked on him daily, and we both transformed. In that time I developed an amazing relationship and trust with Spirit. I made a personal commitment to Spirit, to move with each directive that I was given. I had been taken from death into life, and my intention was to continue to commit more and more to living.

My life became filled with living. I began working with other people, and the energy—my energy—began to expand. My heart opened more, and more. My marriage began to crumble as I began to change. My husband had married a needy, closed person, and I was not that person anymore. I was alive, healthy, and happy. My marriage ended.

My life was full with my three children and my work with people. I was happy and felt fulfilled. I loved my home, and I had a good, simple life.

My connection to the natural forces was growing, and I was becoming aware of the connection and life force of nature, realizing that I, too, was a part of this wonderful world of nature and that there was no separation between me and the natural forces. I started to become initiated into the shamanic world, understanding my place within that world. I began taking my place. My healing accelerated on many different levels as I began to receive understanding about my life and my journey up to this point, and as I began to forgive myself and resurrect myself.

I was guided by Spirit to go on a vision quest, a journey in nature for a weekend, to deepen my alliance with nature and the natural forces. It was here that I had my first vision. The sun was rising, and as it rose it began to spin, creating shafts of brilliant light. The light began to form into a gigantic spider web. In the very center of the web was a light, brilliant and expanded. It pulsated into me, and it came with a message. I was told I must leave Australia in one month's time, leave my children, and go to live in America. I was only to take one suitcase with me. The vision was so strong and dramatic I could not deny the message, as much as I wanted to.

Leave my children! I couldn't imagine walking away from them, and yet I knew that it was right, and that it was something I had to do. I didn't know how I would do it, or how I could do it!

I was told I must tell my children within 48 hours that I was going.

This was the next step for me. I had committed to trust Spirit; I had promised to move with my guidance. I knew I was more and more being taken into being alive—that there was a mission I had to fulfill. I didn't understand or know what that was, but the feeling was so strong, it was as though my heart was being torn in two and there was nothing I could do but move forward. America was my next step.

I was truly afraid but I kept receiving the message: "Don't let the fear stop you, it's only a feeling!" This did not help with the deep pain I was feeling in my heart. I knew that my children would never look at me the same way again once I told them.

I sent my two youngest boys to live with their father; my daughter had a job and was old enough to be by herself. It was a very difficult time. My children were angry; my friends judged me for leaving my children. I was very alone and really afraid. I didn't know anyone in America. I didn't know where I was to go, or what I was to do there. All I could do was keep coming back to the rightness of it, as hard as it was. I had to trust.

The only way I got on to the airplane was to tell my mind that if I didn't like it I could come back in a week. The fear was intense. I had some clarity on booking my ticket to San Francisco, and had seen a course on Light Body being held soon after my arrival. I had called and booked myself into the course, which was being held in Mt. Shasta. I thought Mt. Shasta was a suburb of San Francisco. The person running the course was kind enough to pick me up at the airport, so on landing in San Francisco I was driven directly up to Mt. Shasta.

I did jump off a cliff leaving my native Australia, but I was so held by Spirit and supported in my journey, finding myself in this amazing place: Mt. Shasta—what an incredible mountain! The energy was extraordinary and the natural forces so powerful, I would receive energy from the mountain daily, and there were powerful energy vortexes that opened up many initiations for me.

I lived in Mt. Shasta for one year, working with people and going through profound initiations and experiences. My energies and work expanded. I began running workshops with groups of people as well as individual sessions. I was busy; I was happy. I loved being on this mountain. In my mind I saw myself living on that mountain forever.

Then I was directed by Spirit to do a retreat for two months: to just sit, open to receive. It was a powerful time for me, and my heart opened and expanded as I aligned more and more to the spiritual energies. I was transported into many different energetic realms and went through many different healing processes. I was given understanding and knowledge throughout this time, and I was deeply touched and grateful. I had to use the reserves of my finances in order to live during that time. Trust!

When the two months were up I had almost no money left, and my children were coming to visit for six weeks. It was wonderful to see them, but my financial reserves were completely gone by the time they were leaving. I drove them to the San Francisco airport and gave them the last of my money as they left.

I had arranged and organized to work with a group of people in the Mill Valley area, so I drove toward there from the airport. I had a map with me with directions to the downtown area where I was going to call so I could be taken to the house where I was going to be working.

I had left myself one quarter to make the call, and had no other money. It was dark and raining by the time I arrived. I found the phone box, put my quarter in, and dialed the number, and nothing happened: The phone was not working, and I lost my quarter.

There I was, stranded in the night, in the rain, with no money and no way of contacting my friend. In that moment I was totally panicked. Everything I had left behind in Australia—my friends, my children, my safe life—gone. I had trusted, and look at where I was: with nothing, lost.

My mind snapped, and something shattered inside me. I was shaking and terrified; my trust gone; everything gone. What a fool I had been taking this path, trusting like that!

I walked slowly back to the car not knowing what to do, feeling complete despair and hopelessness. As I got back into the car I noticed something on the floor of the car. The streetlight from above was shining on something. I reached down and there on the floor was another quarter!

This made me laugh. I made the call to my friend and began another level of my work.

It was a turning point for me, and from then on my life and work accelerated. I was never in that same place again. The shattering was a part of my ego letting go, and I came to understand that without that intense experience in that moment I could not have had the healing I needed, or been able to move to another place within myself.

My youngest son joined me after my first year in America, and it was wonderful to have him with me. I was teaching the work to groups of people, continuing to unfold with Spirit, and still moving with the directives given to me by Spirit. I was busy channeling in the new aspects of the work in order to teach the first body of work that had been given to me.

My relationship to the light, to Spirit, was my main focus. I continued to commit to living and moving in alignment with the light—my light. I was continually being taken into deeper aspects of my light, experiencing a deeper union with the light, which was opening me up to many initiations to my Self. I was being moved into a new clarity of truth and healing that was so beautiful, and being opened up to so much knowledge and understanding of my path and mission here on this earth plane.

All that I knew was that I was being guided by the light—by God. My thoughts were uncomplicated on who or what was taking me. I just let go and moved with trust. I would be asked, "Do you work with your guides?" and I would say, "I am guided by the light, and I have wonderful experiences of God." I was very grateful for my journey. I didn't understand why I had been chosen to do this work, but I was committed and honored, and as the work unfolded more and more I found it a humbling experience. It's as though the work and I had become one.

Every day I would walk in a very sacred place near my home. I was called to be in nature, and received a blessing each day in this sacred place. I knew every tree and every rock, and I loved the relationship that I had with this place. I would generally go each morning to see the sun rise and walk the path. It was filled with energetic vortexes and dimensional doorways. Sometimes I would enter these energetic spaces and sometimes just walk by them. I was always so guided by this place.

One day as I entered my sacred walk I became aware of something very different. I entered a world that I had never experienced. There was a group of Alien beings—Pleiadians—waiting to receive me. I was shocked. I didn't believe in spaceships and Aliens! The energy was pure light—love being directed toward me. They were greeting me, gathering me toward them, embracing me. Suddenly I was opened up. I gasped as my consciousness expanded and came into a full remembrance of my Pleiadian heritage: my life simultaneously lived with the Pleiadians and my life here on the earth plane. I found myself moving into my full Pleiadian self. I looked down at Christine, as I came into the full memory of my mission here on this earth plane, choosing this mission, and my Pleiadian life and family. I was standing and experiencing my full light in this Pleiadian consciousness.

I don't know how long I was there in that place with my other family, but I found myself back at my house with no memory of how I got home. I was in an incredible state of expansion.

I was thrown into a deeply disturbed place. I could not discount my experience; it was too powerful. However, I did not want to be a Pleiadian. I did not want this information. I did not want this truth. I was terribly confused and disorientated. Expanded light was pulsating in my body. It was so extreme that I could barely move, and I felt totally without any form. I was just aware of being a radiating energy; I had lost my sense of my physical body. I did not have any sensory experiences of my body: I could not feel the wind on my face; I could not feel the warmth of the sun. All I was experiencing was this extreme light—a blinding light, day and night. I could not rest in the intensity of this experience. I was deeply distressed in this state as this brilliant, blinding light continued to pulse into me.

I remained this way for two months, hardly able to function, and at the same time reeling from the truth of what had taken place and the truth of who I was. I was angry. I didn't know how to continue in my life with this truth. I wanted to go back to how I was before; I didn't want this! There was such conflict going on inside of me; I didn't know how to bring the two pieces together: my connection to God and my Pleiadian self.

Gradually I came to the realization of the love that was present in my Self, and I was given the understanding that there is only the oneness and the Pleiadians are part of that oneness—part of the whole—and that I am part of that whole—the God consciousness. I awakened to the simple truth of oneness of all things.

The work that had come through me many years ago was from the Pleiadians, though I would have been unable to cope with this truth at the time. Now I could deal with it, now that I had such a strong connection to the light and had built a strong anchoring of truth within me. I had to embrace this truth, and to live this truth. It was part of my destiny. I couldn't deny the truth of what was going on. I knew it was true, and I needed to move forward with this truth. I emerged from this experience stronger, and very aware of my Pleiadian family surrounding me in incredible love. I was to become an important link between the Pleiadians and the initiation work they were bringing here to anchor on this earth plane for humankind.

It would take six years before I was fully able to integrate the full energy of my Pleiadian self into my human form. My work expanded into Israel, where I began to teach regularly and work extensively with children.

I was drawn to the Galilee area in Israel, to Capernaum, which is on the Sea of Galilee. Capernaum is the city that was formed for Jesus. I had a strong guidance to go there, although I had not previously had any particular relationship to Jesus. I had no religious background or interaction with his energy. The pull to go there was intense.

As I arrived and I got out of the car I was overcome with emotion— emotion so strong that it brought me to my knees. I was on the ground sobbing uncontrollably, as though my heart was tearing open, not with grief but with an intense joy. It was birthing right through my heart. I was on the ground for an hour, completely overcome. I didn't know how I was going to actually walk into this place, and take in the energy there.

Suddenly I felt Jesus with me. He asked me to walk down to the edge of the Sea of Galilee and just stand there. I walked down to the sea. It was beautiful and calming. I stood there trying to collect myself, feeling a peace inside me. As I looked out across the water I saw a form coming toward me. It was Jesus walking across the water toward me, with his arms outstretched and light flowing all around him. The love was so strong it was pulsing through me, and the light that was sur- rounding him was coming into me and surrounding me. He came and placed his hands on the top of my head and I felt an incredible anoint- ing. He then took my hands in his, and we walked together along the shoreline. He talked to me about love and referred to my ministry with people, and the importance of the teaching and action of love.

Jesus is a constant teacher in my life and continues to help me with so much love. He has taught me so much about loving myself with compassion. He told me his main mission here is love—that we as human beings have come here to take ourselves off the cross, and to resurrect ourselves. My journey with Jesus has been life changing. He has given me clarity on what love truly is and how that energy of pure love can transform everything. He has given me the opportunity of healing, helping me to understand myself and my life, so that I have been able to open to a true compassion, and the true self-loving principal that I so badly needed for me to receive myself back.

I received a channeled directive to begin teaching the second body of work that I had been given those many years ago. I was told that the earth plane was now ready for these initiations that were activated by the Frequencies of Brilliance work. This brought me into a deeper and more active role with the Pleiadians as I began teaching and transmitting this initiating work.

The Frequencies of Brilliance work expanded me quickly into many new levels of awareness of myself and the experience of the work was beautiful. As my energy expanded, my work expanded in the world. It flowed out to Brussels, Holland, Italy, Canada, Brazil, and Argentina, and throughout the United States. Everything began accelerating in my world as I initiated people into this new work. It was an honor to bring this pure initiation to the planet and work even more closely with the Pleiadians.

Sai Baba is a teacher and a friend who has played a powerful role in my life. He has taught me the power of laughter, and not to take myself too seriously. I love the fact that he is on this earth plane in the physical form, and has the ability to appear to me anywhere at any time. Sometimes he has called me to come to him at the ashram in Puttaparti. He says, "It's time for you to come and be in my place for a while." My heart is filled with gratitude for his constant presence in my life.

I first connected to him in 1985. I had just read a book about him and about four hours later he appeared in my bedroom and said, "It's time to come to see me in India." I was shocked, and said to him, "That's impossible!"

He said, "The way will be made clear." And he disappeared.

I had no money, and if I had money it certainly wouldn't be to go to India!

About three weeks later my best friend's father, who thought of me as a daughter, gave me $4,000, with the instruction it was only to be used for myself. Four weeks later I was in the ashram at Puttaparti. I was there for a month, at the hottest time of the year, in the high desert in the south of India with high winds and dust flying. I hated it!

My anger and misery grew day by day. By the time I left I was fully enraged. It was as if all the rage that had been locked inside me loosened. As I left I heard Sai Baba say to me, "You will return." And I said, "Never!"

It was two months after returning home that I was diagnosed with lupus. I know now that the emotional energy that was released at the ashram opened up my next step. I was not to have another conscious experience with Sai Baba for 12 years. I have been to his Ashram four more times during the last 13 years. They were very different visits from my first trip, but of course I had transformed in consciousness by the second visit. And I have been extremely privileged to have his support in my work. He continues to teach me in my life.

I was given the guidance to go to Bosnia. I was told to go to Medjogoria, which is where Mother Mary has appeared to many people. There is a mountain where thousands of people come for healing. They walk up the mountain, and it is there that many people have experienced the apparition of Mother Mary. Many have experienced miraculous healing in this place.

When I arrived in Medjogoria I walked along the streets of the town. There was so much despair and desolation showing in people's faces. There had been terrible war, and the people and place seemed shattered.

I walked the streets in the freezing cold wind. I could not get warm; the wind was so strong and cold there was hardly anyone on the streets, and certainly no pilgrims around to walk up the mountain on that day. The sky was really black. It was mid-morning but with the heavy dark sky it felt more like evening.

I received a message. I was to go up on the mountain. I was not impressed and had a huge resistance, but of course I had to go. My commitment was to follow my guidance no matter what! I dressed as warmly as I could. The wind howled as I began the long, steep climb up the mountain. I was alone on the path. The higher I climbed the colder and windier it got. I battled the wind. I kept being pushed back by its incredible strength. The sky was getting darker and darker. I was getting angrier and angrier, and fed up. The wind was getting stronger and stronger, and colder and colder.

When I reached the top it was terrible; conditions were worse, and the only way I could prevent myself from being blown off the mountain was to crouch inside the base of this huge metal cross that stands at the very top of the mountain. I crawled inside the cross, into the base, and rested there, protecting myself from the wind, still freezing cold, and thinking to myself, "What am I doing here? This is crazy!"

Suddenly there was a light in the sky, as though the black clouds parted a little and let in this glorious light. I looked up and saw Mother Mary. The light came shining down into me, and I was filled with warmth and a great love. Mother Mary spoke to me about the importance of my mission here on earth and of the work I was to do in the world, but there was something more important than all the work I had to do—and that was me. I was the most important focus, and she told me she was here to support *me,* not the work. It was her job to support and love me on my journey in this lifetime. She asked me to open myself up to her, and call upon her at any time and she would be there.

Tears rolled down my face. It was hard to put the focus on me, and to believe that I was worthy of this gift of love. I had never known a mother's love, and she gave me that. It was many years before I was able to fully receive that from her, and take in the grace that I had been given on that day. The light disappeared and I was back into the blackness and in the howling wind. Inside me I was warm and filled with the light from Mother Mary. It was a difficult journey back down the mountain against the wind, but I was so filled with Mary's warmth it made the journey easy. She held me as I made my way back down the mountain.

Mary has been with me ever since, always by my side when I call to her. I could never have guessed how much of a role she was going to play in my healing process connected to my childhood. Without her I do not think I would have been able to deal with healing the huge wounds that were inside of me.

A few years later, I was present at the birth of my first grandchild. I was unprepared for the incredible joy that birthed through my heart, as she was born. The birth activated a deep process within me—a deep process within my heart. It's as though something in my heart opened for the first time, a new vulnerability as I held my granddaughter for the first time. The joy and connection that I felt with her was magical and deep, allowing a new opening to take place within my heart.

On returning home that vulnerability deepened, to the point that I felt I needed rest. I didn't understand what was happening. There was a feeling of being out of control and completely exposed. I was so distracted by this experience that later in the day as I was closing the garage I jammed three of my fingers in the garage door. The pain was extreme, and I experienced a shocking terror running through my body. It was such an intense feeling, and yet, strangely, a very familiar feeling at the same time.

At the hospital I could not stop crying, and I didn't know why I could not stop crying. But my heart was aching and I was feeling so afraid, almost in terror of something. All three fingers were broken, and the doctor told me that I would need three weeks of rest to heal them.

The feelings inside continued to accelerate, and I was plummeted into experiences I didn't understand. I felt as though my sense of reality was gone, and the feelings of terror and being out of control escalated. I realized that this had something to do with my past, my childhood, and I needed help. I began to realize that I was somehow flashing back to my past, though these memories were new, and the feelings and experiences felt like they were happening to me now.

I prayed to find a therapist who could help me navigate through the maze of flashbacks. I was given a miracle and found a therapist who specialized in cult-ritual abuse victims. I flew to Los Angeles to work with her. After two days of therapy she said, "Things will probably get a lot worse before they get better." She was right.

This was the beginning of the return of the memories of the incredible nightmare of my childhood. My family of origin was involved in a cult, and in this I was subjected to many abuses and traumatic practices as a child. My mother had polio when I was a year old. She became a cripple for the rest of her life, and I became the scapegoat for her pain and rage. She looked at me as the cause of her polio. If I had not been born, she would have been all right. A deal was made between my parents and the cult: I was to be given to the cult to play a part in their many rituals in return for my mother's healing. At home I was part of a sexual triangle with my mother and my father, so my life was taken over by these many traumatic experiences, and I became hopelessly lost to myself.

These memories accelerated and totally took over my life for the next three to four years. I lived with flashbacks, reliving one horrible experience after another. For a period of time I was totally out of control and lived in constant terror. I had to move to Los Angeles to be near my therapist, and I stopped work for three months in order to have therapy 16 hours a week. The only time I could leave my apartment was to get to therapy; the rest of the time I was in terror as I worked my way through the maze of horror. I just wanted it to be over. I was forced to feel what I had buried deep inside me—buried so deep so that I could survive. I wished for death, and I remember wishing for death as a child.

This process of healing seemed endless, but through it all Mother Mary was with me, giving me the support and the courage to open up to such tremendous pain and suffering. She held each internal child part, and opened up the possibility of me being able to reach out to these parts of myself that had split off in order to survive the horror of what we had lived through in the cult. I cannot believe how held I was through this nightmare. The Angels surrounded me and kept me safe through the darkest times.

My belief as a child that I was alone—so completely abandoned—changed as I began to resurrect myself. As I came back to the memories I was shown that the Angels had been there with me through all the dreadful experiences. But I had chosen to close off as a child, so I could just survive. I wasn't able to experience the help that was there for me at the time.

As I continued my therapy healing happened; miracles happened. With my therapist's help I navigated myself through the layers of memory that surfaced with the pain, guilt, grief, and rage. I began to connect to a new part of myself, and to experience and connect to the inner children. These were the most courageous parts of myself: the inner kids who took on the most painful, the most shocking experiences that I went through. Without these parts doing this, I never would have survived my ordeal.

So as I resurrected these child parts of myself I began to heal, and then more of me became available. I began to feel more secure within myself in the world, and more stable and complete within my world. I could feel myself coming back to life, so that I was able just to feel more, to feel more joy in my life, to be more present in every moment, and to be more connected to my life. I was able to be more a part of what was going on in the world around me in my day-to-day life. I was much less afraid, and more able to cope with being in the world. I began to develop an understanding of myself, and how I was really feeling in each moment: much more honest with myself, and with my feelings that were present. I began to feel free and to be more authentically *me*. It was a great feeling to be able to depend on myself and to know how I was feeling, and no longer be a victim, reacting to the external world. I was be able to depend on myself to be stable.

It was good to be able to connect and understand my kid parts inside of me, and to be able to move out of the longtime separation that had taken place within me. I could depend on myself to take care of me, and to hold the kid parts inside so that a healing relationship was able to take place between me and my kids. I had to become the parent to them, giving them stability and love, and as I did this it allowed the inner kids to begin to grow. As they began to feel safe and listened to, they began to trust me to be there for them. As they began to trust me they began to experience a resurrection, to be able to move away from the pain of the past, and then be able to be here in the present life that we were living, and feeling held in a safe loving place.

My kids brought me back into connecting to an innocent part of me. Through their eyes I could experience the world differently. They brought me into a world of wonderment, and a new appreciation of the beauty of nature and the joy of life.

There was much more of me available now. A new authentic part of me was emerging, and as I emerged my connection to the spiritual realms increased. My channel was clearer and so my communicating skills with the Pleiadians, Spirit, and the Natural forces increased. I felt as though a huge burden was being lifted off me. I was actually lifting it off myself, as I resurrected into a new understanding and truth for myself. Me resurrecting me.

I am forever grateful, for the help from Mother Mary throughout that time. I could never have taken these steps alone, and there were so many miracles connected to my healing and the never-ending love from Mother Mary.

When I finally returned to work I could feel a new sense of connection to myself and my connection to Spirit. Times were still not easy, though when I was working I was in perfect alignment with Spirit and the Pleadians; when I finished work I was back dealing with parts of myself that were still healing. There were still fear and some flashbacks, and I had to continue to commit to my full healing and continue moving through my process. Not easy. I would work with my therapist by phone as I traveled with work, and when I was back at home I continued therapy for 12 hours a week. My healing process went on for the next four years. I am doing much better. I have been able to move out of Los Angeles and, when I am home, I speak with my therapist once a week.

This healing process has been profound. I continue to experience a deeper sense of freedom and a deep connection with myself inside. My inner kids and I have been reunited, and I am so grateful for my healing.

Dealing with this part of my past was the hardest thing I have ever done, and I believe that I could not have dealt with it before that time. It was my strong connection to Mother Mary, Spirit, and the Pleiadians that made it possible for me to go into the very depth of hell to find these inner kid parts, and resurrect myself. Without these alliances, I would not have been able to open up to meet these memories and the deep trauma that was inside of me.

In June 2008, I was working in a monastery near Banneux, which is a sacred site where Mother Mary had appeared many times to a young girl in 1933. A small community had built up in the area where the many apparitions had taken place. I was strongly drawn to Banneux, and every afternoon after finishing work I would walk to the sanctuary where I could strongly feel the presence of Mary. Every day I was drawn like a magnet into the different areas where she had appeared long ago. Mary would greet me with so much love each time I would go, and my heart was deeply touched by each encounter. I didn't fully understand what was taking place with these experiences but I knew I was in the middle of some important and deep transformational processes with her. She kept reminding me that she was here to support me in the different phases of my journey and would always be there for me. I was not a stranger to these experiences with her, as I had many encounters with her energies in Israel and in Medjagoria. She had always appeared to me at critical junctions in my life.

After the first three days of going to see her I could feel my heart expanding, more and more. I went to sleep on the third night of being with her, and some time later in the night awoke to find that I was outside of my body. I was trying to get back into my body, but I couldn't. I was disoriented and confused. Why couldn't I get back into my body? I reached out and touched my body and it was icy cold. What was going on? What was happening? I felt a panic run through me as I suddenly realized that my body was no longer breathing. I was dead!

I felt as though something slammed into me in that moment. I couldn't breathe—couldn't think. Nothing I knew made sense and I began to spiral into a total panic. Suddenly Mary appeared beside me, her light and warmth calming me immediately. She told me I had completed everything I had come here to achieve; I had completed all my personal transformations that I had set for myself in this lifetime. I had just completed it much earlier than expected, and my life was now over.

She was so calm and matter-of-fact about my situation, stating it without drama. But I was so upset, distraught by this news. I wanted to go back; I wasn't ready to leave my life! Something had to be done. I told her of my need to be here on the planet in this life, and in this body, and the work that I still had to complete. I asked her to help me to go back.

She explained that once a blueprint is completed, life is over for that person. You cannot be on the earth plane without an active blueprint. Each person who comes here to the earth plane creates an energetic blueprint for themselves before they come into their lives. This blueprint contains what they intend to achieve within themselves here in their lifetime. In order for me to go back into my body and continue my life I would have to create a new blueprint for myself for this lifetime.

I agreed to create a new blueprint for myself. Mary held me in her arms and I felt like a newborn child. She held me with love as I opened up to the energy to create my new blueprint. As I did this I was filled with Mary's light and compassion. I could feel a new life force filling me, and a new energy of myself opening up through consciousness. The new blueprint was completed, and I was in a deep state of union with Mother Mary. She told me I could now re-enter my physical body and to place my hands on my chest. I re-entered my body and placed my hands on my chest. I felt a life force move through all my cells as my body came alive again. There was such relief to be back in my body, and back in my life. I felt so much gratitude for my life, so much joy for being alive. I had never realized how much I needed to be here and how important it was for me to be on this earth plane at this time. Every day I am filled with the same gratitude that I felt in that moment of coming back into my body: another chance to be here, and to live more consciously.

Two days later I was in the middle of my workday when suddenly Mother Mary appeared to me. She had her hands up toward me, and her energy was flowing from them into me. I was filled with a tremendous love and peace, and at the same time I could feel an adjustment of energy inside my body, as though I could take a breath for the first time since my experience two days earlier. Her love just held me, and then she disappeared. She reappeared two consecutive days, each time transmitting a light into me and then disappearing. Each time I felt another level of energy integrating through my cells, though emotionally I was still reeling inside from the experience.

Many months passed and I moved further away from my experience until I was no longer conscious of having had the experience at all. It was as though it never took place. Then one day a close friend with whom I had shared this experience reconnected with me. The first thing he asked me was, "How have you been since your death experience?" I was shocked by his words, and it brought the experience back into me as though it had just taken place. My mind began to panic as I relived that moment of no longer being alive. I then realized how deeply traumatized I had been. I began to gently re-examine my feelings from that time, and allow myself to feel the depth of them. As I did this I began to comprehend the importance of my death experience. I was able to feel myself and the vulnerability that came into me when my heart expanded with Mary. It was when she held me, when I birthed my new blueprint, that I moved into a deeper place within my own heart. I had created the blueprint through my Sacred heart, the most expanded place within my heart, and in that moment, it moved me to another place within myself.

Which part of me decided to create it? What did I create in my new blueprint? I opened up to go back and revisit the full experience, which was difficult—to feel the depth of my vulnerability during the creation of my blueprint. I knew instantly that it involved an expanded opening of my Sacred heart. My light and my consciousness were able to move into this opening of my heart in that moment and I began to experience a new depth of connection to all levels of consciousness.

As I did this I was then able to open up to the information that had been waiting for me to be able to receive. I consciously opened up to my heart and said, "Yes, I am ready to open to this truth in my experience. I am ready to feel!"

As I consciously opened back up to the experience I could see brilliant blue light expanding down into my physical body, effervescent in form and filled with diamond-shaped lights. These forms filled my body, and as they entered me there was a blending of energy through me. This blending created deep energetic connections to the multi-dimensional aspects of my Self.

In this moment my conscious Self re-birthed into my form. This began to align me into a deep truth and understanding of my new mission for the rest of this lifetime, to the details of my new blueprint. My heart began to consciously connect into the energy of my mission. I was given a deeper reconnection to the loving aspect to the unique divine aspect of myself. I felt so much grace in that moment.

I consciously opened to my transformation and the truth of all that I am now, of all that I said *yes* to. It was like reclaiming myself consciously in that moment, and a consolidation of my experience began to take place through my spiritual, physical, and emotional body. I began to understand why I had needed time to take my death experience into my consciousness. The deep vulnerability that was opened up during the experience was too much for me to accept and be with. I needed time to process the depth of it and allow myself to digest the energetic changes first.

I know now that this new vulnerability created a new strength within me. It opened my heart to a new level of compassion, and gave me a deeper access to Universal truth and an understanding of that truth. I live each day with a new level of awareness of the light and a consciousness of my place within that, working with this consciousness as a true part of the oneness—the whole. My whole world has transformed for me and continues to open up more each day.

Exactly one year after this experience happened, I was back in Belguim, working about one hour away from Banneux. I was drawn back to the sacred site and spent the afternoon with Mother Mary at the many sacred places where she appeared. It was a gift to be back in this place and to experience once more her loving presence and energy with me as I walked through the different areas of Banneux. She stayed very close to me during that week as I celebrated the anniversary of my death experience—actually, to be more accurate, my new life experience!

It is an amazing thing to be able now to be so aligned and part of the Universal consciousness on a completely new level; to move through the world with my resurrected heart; and to feel the depth of all things. My gratitude grows daily as I continue to unfold into myself.

I continue my journey day-by-day committing to each moment of life, knowing that life is truly the teacher, and I can rest knowing that I am being shown the truth in each moment. It is with great gladness and appreciation that I live this life now.

So be it!

Working With the Inner Child

I want to bring to your attention an important aspect of yourself that needs to be addressed as you work within the Pleiadian chapters of this book. Know that, in order for you to open up more completely to this new level of yourself, you need to have a working relationship with your inner child. Your journey to Self cannot be completed without this conscious connection to your child within. The connection to your child is very supportive in the journey with your initiations with the Pleiadians. I want to talk about the inner child so that you can open up to or expand your existing relationship to the child inside you.

Some of you had a wonderful, healthy childhood; you were loved and nurtured. But there are many of you who had a difficult childhood, perhaps with very traumatic events or many abuses taking place. It is irrelevant which type of childhood you experienced. What is important is that you begin to connect to your inner child and/or expand the connection that you already have. You need the energy of that child in your life, and that child needs this connection to you.

No one has a perfect childhood; there are always events and experiences that affect you, and some of those things still affect you today. There are triggers from that time in your childhood that operate in your day-to-day lives as an adult, in your personal relationships, in the way you bring up your own children, and in the way you interact with other people.

The reason it is so important to have a relationship with your inner child with these initiations is that as you open up to these initiating energies you begin to transform. You begin to move out of separation, aligning more completely with your light Self, which moves you increasingly into your place within the Universal Consciousness, and into the Oneness. You cannot fully move into your place within these spaces while you are separate from your inner child. There needs to be a healing—a coming together with you and your inner child.

You will find that, as your relationship deepens with your child, you merge, and together you will move through each initiation process. The child holds an innocence and purity that will help you in your journey home: back to yourself. I cannot stress enough how important it is.

I am eternally grateful to my inner kids for the courage they had, to hold so much of my past pain. Now they show me a new world with their innocence, joy, and love. I came to realize that I needed this aspect of myself. It brought much more balance to my life and allowed me to connect more strongly to the love that exists here within this universe. It allowed me to not feel alone on this planet.

As you realign with the inner child you will find that your world will be more flowing, and you will have more clarity about what is going on around you and how you feel. You will feel more complete, more relaxed, and whole.

Let's talk about the childhood process: how the child thinks and operates in the world.

As children we think we are in control—that we are responsible for everything that happens around us and to us. It's what I call "magic thinking." The reason children think this way is because in reality children are completely vulnerable: dependent upon the adults around them to take care of them and to give them love. So the child thinks this way so that he or she will be in control, but in reality, as children, we are anything but in control. Every child needs love, and in the quest for love children quickly discover what they need to do and how they need to act to get that love.

In a healthy relationship with parents this is not such a problem. But in unhealthy relationships we, as children, learn to do whatever we need to do to get love. When we don't get the love, we think, "I must just not be good enough," or "There must be something wrong with me."

If the parents fight, if the parents are angry, if the parents separate, or if the parents physically abuse the child, the child feels "If only I had been good enough this would not have happened," or "This is my fault." The child personalizes what is taking place around him or her. The child feels responsible, and by feeling responsible the child also feels in control. It is safer to feel in control than helpless, because being helpless creates too much pain. You cannot survive with helplessness, so in order to survive the child takes full responsibility for everything that happens. The child feels responsible for the angry parent, sad parent, or abusive parent. The responsibility then creates incredible guilt, shame, and self-loathing.

As we grow into adults we bring with us these issues from childhood, locked inside with our inner child, and affecting our lives and our relationships with others. We may isolate ourselves, not letting other people into our personal space. We make sure we are alone, and safe. Or we may be in an abusive relationship that doesn't give us the love we need. Or we may be the abuser in the relationship. We may recreate physical abuse in our relationship, or we may even become our own abuser. We tend to pattern our adult relationships on what took place in our relationships with our parents or caregivers, unless we get help to break the cycle.

Your past will also affect the way that you take care of yourself now, how much you allow yourself to have in the way of physical comfort, and what you provide for yourself in terms of enough rest and relaxation—how you nutritionally feed your physical body. Some of the pain can be expressed by driving yourself constantly: always working, never giving yourself time to rest, never really giving yourself any loving attention. It will affect the way you can receive love and the way you can allow yourself to just be in the world.

Each one of us has a child inside of us. It is up to us to reach inside and connect with that child. As you do this, your child will come forward to meet you. You can do this; it is about resurrecting a lost part of yourself.

Let's talk about another process that takes place when there is a lot of abuse and/or trauma in your childhood years. When the pain and fear are too great to deal with when we are children, the child parts split off. One part of the child holds the pain and the experience of fear, so that the other part of your child can survive. Some of us as adults have more than one child part. In order to heal and bring back these child parts that are holding the past trauma, you need to be able to open up and access the child who is holding the memory from that time. Allow that child part to be able to feel the feelings that are connected with the incidents from the past.

I call it resurrecting the child because, while this child part is still holding the pain, this inner child part is hiding deep inside of you. The only reality this child part inside of you has is the past, so that part is constantly in fear, and time has frozen so the child part is unaware that you are now an adult and your life has changed. The only way you ever experience this inner child part is when an incident takes place in your life that mirrors some aspect of the time as a child when the trauma played out. It could be a smell, music, or the sound of a voice; it could be a person who reminds you of someone who was part of the trauma; it could be a similar emotion that is coming up inside of you that mirrors your past trauma.

The first thing to understand when you are moving toward that child in crisis is that the only important element toward healing is moving toward the feeling—to access the feeling of the child inside you. To do this you need to first begin to establish trust between you and the child.

Trust can only be established if you are willing to be consistent with them, following through on promises and giving them a little time each day—maybe 10 minutes to begin with, so you can establish a connection and relationship with them.

To begin with you can just talk to the child inside, explain that you want to reconnect with him or her, and ask the child to come and be with you. Walking in nature and sharing the flowers with the child, the birds, looking up at the sky—all these things are a good way to begin to connect to the child. Drawing is also a great way for the child to have time to connect to you. Let him or her choose a color crayon and draw; let the child have an avenue to express him- or herself. The child will respond to you; just be consistent and patient.

As you do this, the child will emerge, and as he or she begins to move toward you, you open to the next step of holding that child. As you hold the child you will begin to connect to the feelings that are there. Some of these feelings will be deep. Let yourself feel and remind the child that he or she is remembering and feeling something that happened a long time ago, and that he or she is very safe now with you. Just keep holding the child part and let the feelings continue to come out.

An important first step is to let the child know that time has moved on, that you are no longer a child, and as an adult you can protect this child inside. Use examples such as where you now live and the difference in your surroundings to where you used to live. Let the child inside know that you will not let anyone hurt him or her again and that you can keep him or her safe.

This is an important healing step. It begins to resurrect an inner part of you, and you are then able to recollect and resurrect parts of yourself. You begin to move into a different type of wholeness. As this wholeness develops and deepens, you feel a new sense of lightness and joy enter your life. For those of you who have had severe abuse in your childhood, this process will likely need the support of a therapist. The reason is that, as the memories surface, you will need a deeper process than the one mentioned previously. As the past trauma begins to surface, there are many layers to be dealt with. For me, there is no way I would have been able, by myself, to navigate through the enormous amount of pain and terror that was locked inside of me.

Resurrection of these child parts is important because you put an end to the separation inside of yourself. It is part of the work we are doing in this book. In your spiritual awakening you are ending separation, rejoining the light aspect of your Self. Each step you take with this child will assist you in each step of your initiations within each chapter.

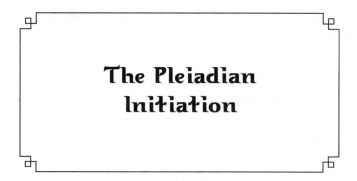

The Pleiadian Initiation

Now it is time to move into the Pleiadian initiations section of this book. Each chapter builds on the previous chapter, so it is advised that you work chapter by chapter, listening to the audio tracks connected to each chapter in their numbered order.

Have a wonderful journey. I honor each one of you as you take this unfolding journey of yourself.

Message From the Pleiadians

My beloved one, we are here to assist you in your alignment back to your natural Self. For lifetimes you have been separated from the whole. Now is the time to come back home, to come back and take your place within the whole. You are needed; you are missed. It's for you to awaken now, awaken into your unique aspect of the divine whole, to take your place.

We have designed this book to energetically initiate you, so that you can re-align yourself back to the Self. We are committed in assisting you, by holding energetic dimensional spaces open while you birth yourself, and open to remembering and aligning yourself to Universal Truth, moving yourself out of the third-dimensional illusions. Resurrecting yourself and aligning yourself back to a fourth/fifth-dimensional reality. It is the time for you, for your planet, to realign. It is an exciting time for you to awaken and remember. It is a process of bringing yourself back into a remembrance of Self. That is why it is called an awakening!

This awakening is being assisted by a new energy that has just begun to be anchored and activated onto this earth plane. It began its transmission on the 1st of January 2009. It is known as the "Self Healing Prophecy." The energy of this Prophecy was always going to be anchored at this time on your planet. Its timing is perfectly aligned to assist you in adjusting to the energetic transition that is taking place here on your planet. We, the Pleiadians, have our part to play in anchoring the many levels of this awakening energy. The new levels will be anchored, as you are ready to receive them. Understand that there are many dimensional layers to the Prophecy's energies. They will be transmitted onto the earth plane in different levels, as you are ready to receive them. The Prophecy's energies are for you individually, and also for the Collective Consciousness of your planet. This involves the energies of the Earth itself, affecting the energetic grid lines that run through the Earth.

What is this energy and what is it here for?

This energy from the Prophecy is a gift that has been given to all of you human beings to assist you in an accelerated awakening of remembering the Truth of yourselves. It is designed to take you into a state of "remembering": Remembering who you are in your spiritual self and your place within the Collective Consciousness in the Universal realms. The Self Healing Prophecy energy is going to help you move into a deeper alignment to your Self, your connection to the higher aspects of you. This is a grace period given to all of you at this time. It has been activated now so there can be a huge shift within the "consciousness" of your planet now. This means that the Prophecy energies are going to activate a lifting of the veils that have been on this planet for lifetimes. With the lifting of the veils you will be able to awaken on a spiritual level, at an accelerated rate. It will bring you into a new alignment with all life force within the universe. You will be consciously connected, more aware of the life force within you, and the life force within each individual. This will bring you into an experience of Oneness with all things, and you will begin to remember your place within the Oneness.

The Self Healing Prophecy will help you access and open up your awareness of the different dimensional realms that exist. This will enable you to begin a realignment process to aspects of your multidimensional Self, reconnecting and initiating yourself back to those aspects. As you begin to open to this conscious reconnection, you are able to realign to, and reclaim, your personal power and integrate this energy into the cells of your body. You will be able to utilize this knowledge and energy in this lifetime, now.

This Self Healing Prophecy is going to anchor deeper dimensional levels of itself as we move into the time frame of the years 2010–2012.

How is the Prophecy's energy designed to assist you in achieving what you came here to do in this lifetime? How can it help you now in your life? Let's talk about the energy of this Prophecy and how it is meant to work within your community and within you as an individual.

One of the main roles of the Self Healing Prophecy is to help end separation on this earth plane. With this energy bringing your awareness back to a direct experience with Oneness, you can consciously live the experience of Oneness here on this earth plane, with each other and all living things. Healing of the separation begins with individuals, first ending the separation within themselves.

As an individual you are now being asked to look within yourself, and open to all the personal judgments that you have toward yourself. The separating factors that keep your heart closed, and don't allow you to receive and flourish. This is a self-punishment through the judgments that you hold against yourself. These judgments cause emotional and physical pain inside of you. It is the time for you to turn back toward yourself, holding yourself with love; to just breathe and let go. Hold yourself in love and compassion for this life that you have lived up to this point. You have done the best that you could in each moment. You have come here to this world to have all sorts of experiences. Mistakes are an important part of these experiences.

You will begin to understand the learning experiences you have received in living your story. We refer to your life as your "story" because that is just what it is, a story that has brought you to all that you are in this moment. But there comes a time to let go of this story. You take some very powerful and important steps when you let go of your story.

You have all have a story, you have all had painful experiences to live out, and one person has not had more than another. Different experiences yes, but not more. This is the time for you to let go of your story and move forward, toward yourself, toward love and compassion for you.

Self-judgments get in the way of the self-loving principal. As you judge yourself you automatically judge others, and the loving principal is closed down. Internal wars begin—energetic wars that close off the love even more—setting up walls, closing others out, and closing yourself out from the love. This creates a feeling of separation, aloneness and despair.

It's time to break down the barriers so that you can receive the energies of the Self Healing Prophecy, receive this gift of yourself, this gift of love.

Your first step is to celebrate yourself, for the life you have lived up to this point and turn toward yourself with love, holding your heart and breathing this in. Hold your life in your consciousness, just as you have lived it, and breathe. You have lived it in the way you needed to. As you turn toward yourself with love celebrating all experiences in your life, you will begin to move out of separation of yourself and into a new alignment within your heart. Keep holding yourself and your life with love and breathing. Be patient. Take your time. Then let go.

As the walls begin to break down it will allow you to begin to utilize the energy of this Prophecy, aligning you with aspects of your natural birthright, which is abundance on all levels. It will open you up to working with your natural state of physical self-healing, and becoming conscious in co-creating your world and co-creating your abundance on all levels. You will begin to align with higher light aspects of your Self, resurrecting yourself from the self-judgment and opening into a new sense of freedom within your life and within your self. The Prophecy energy is designed to awaken you into a new lightness of spirit and a new sense of yourself within the world and within the Universal Consciousness.

The Prophecy accelerates your ability to move into a new awareness of your role on this planet and the support that is here for you within the Universe. As you awaken to the truth of your alignment and place within this Universal Consciousness, you can open up to the unlimited aspects of Self that link you into a deep understanding and knowledge of your place within the whole. The energies will move you deeper into a state of Oneness, back to the truth of yourself, and the unconditional love that exists within this connection.

As you open to this truth the love creates openness toward all people in your world. Your heart will be able to transform itself with these new energies, and you will begin to work from your Sacred heart. Your compassionate heart will begin to transmit the love out. You will begin to feel a true connection to other people through your heart. These heart connections are important. They are needed for the awakening of all human beings, for the soul connections, and the soul groups that will be coming together. The Prophecy energies will assist soul groups to find each other. The Prophecy energy is also designed for you to become more aligned with the Spiritual energies in a new way, with a deeper and more conscious connection, so you can work in partnership with Spirit and the energetic realms. The Spirit will help you realign yourself to your energetic blueprint, which you created for yourself before you came to his planet to live your life. It is your mission.

As the inner war with yourself changes, the inner wars with other people in your life also change. The separation ends and love takes its place. Your world is going to transform with this conscious love growing.

As the love begins to grow with yourself and others, Spirit will begin to take your place and feel your place within your world, within your universe, and be able to consciously utilize the help and support that is here for you.

We, the Pleiadians, play an important role with you as you begin to work with this Self Healing Prophecy energy. This book holds many initiating journeys for you that will align you to the Prophecy. We commit to working with you as you navigate yourself on this journey, with your permission.

This is a destiny call for you. You were always going to take this journey, and we were always going to be there to support you. This is our contract; it is a contract of love. The online audio tracks hold the healing frequencies of the "Self Healing Prophecy," which will assist you in with your awakening energies so that you can move forward into oneness and your place within the Universal grid much more easily. It is for you to call us forward as you wish to have our assistance in your process. We totally honor your individual process, and your right to create your journey as you need it to be for you, moment by moment, step by step.

Hold yourself with love as you take these steps.

With Love and Blessings
The Pleiadians

Chapter 1
Connecting to
the Heart

It is through your heart that you will begin to align to the guidance of your Self and to the light of the Self. It is through the heart that you will be able to link into guidance for your journey. This chapter is designed to connect you to your heart and the energy of your heart, and, most important, to the flow of the light of the Self. This flow connects you to the Universal Consciousness and your place within it.

You are going to begin to build a new relationship with your heart. Up to this point most of your connection has been with the mind. Your ego mind has been your guide in your life, controlling your every action. The problem with this is that the ego mind is incredibly limited; it is motivated to keep you in *survival* mode. When you are in survival mode the full motivation connected to decision-making is through fear, lack, and struggle, and these motivations are entirely connected into the illusion of third-dimensional reality. There is no true creativity and freedom in this connection, so the ego mind keeps you in a cycle of limitation and stagnation.

When you listen to the mind, you cannot connect to the guidance of the light of the Self. It means that for you to truly move into your heart connection you cannot afford to allow the ego mind to control your every movement and make the decisions. The ego is like a small child that requires discipline and boundaries. It does not recognize the truth; it does not understand the truth. The ego mind is totally fear-based, and will move you away from anything that it believes to be risky, so that you are constantly limited in your ability to create.

To align to the truth you must be connected to the heart, which is aligned to the light of the Self. To move forward on your path you need to be prepared to trust your heart and flow. You can trust your heart to take you to where you need to go because it's directly connected to the light of the Self. When you connect to the heart and live through the heart you are automatically being taken care of in each moment because you are being guided by the light of your higher Self. You can trust this guidance to take care of you. This is truly taking back your power!

Your heart connection moves you into a place of feeling, and feeling creates healing on the physical, emotional, and spiritual levels. As you begin to feel what is in your heart you begin to move into the present moment, asking yourself, *"What am I feeling now?"* As the feelings come up and the heart begins to expand, you become more alive and more connected to your heart.

Feelings are a key to most of your experiences. If you are willing to open up to the feeling as the experience is taking place, and then take a breath, you will find that the experience itself will lessen in intensity because you are connecting into the feeling. When you connect into the heart you experience the clarity of the moment, and a new understanding.

So stop and take a breath into your heart when there is a difficult situation. Slow yourself down. Take a moment to be present with yourself. When a difficult situation arises, don't leave yourself. Breathe and feel.

As you connect to and clear the emotional pain that has been held in your heart you are able to connect more completely to the *joy* inside, which is a part of who you are. When you suppress the pain, you automatically suppress the joy. You have come here to experience joy and the wonders that are here on this earth plane; to connect to other human beings through the heart; and to experience a sacred union with all living things. Your heart needs to come alive in order to have those experiences. This is what being alive is about: feeling and being a part of all life force and experiencing true passion.

True living is *feeling*—feeling and breathing, through the heart, connecting naturally to the light of the Self, taking your place, and allowing yourself to be held in truth and love, within your place in the universal consciousness. When your heart begins to open you begin to be able to fully receive, and then you can open up to your natural birthright of abundance on all levels.

Once you are in the natural flow of your own light everything in your everyday life changes. There is no struggle, and you move freely in your day-to-day living. There is an inner feeling of calm. It's almost as though you were swimming upstream against the current, and suddenly now you are free flowing downstream, effortlessly. This change is you moving into your natural flow of the light of the Self, and connecting into a natural loving aspect of yourself.

Building the Heart Muscle

Human beings say that they want to remember—to know their path, and to find out why they are here and what their mission is in this lifetime. *What am I doing here? What is the purpose of my life?*

To really connect to the answers to these questions you are going to have to change *where* you look for direction in your life and where you connect to receive those answers. Then you can receive the truth to your questions. Then you can move in an alignment to your Self in your life. You will only receive the answers to these questions from within yourself, and these answers can be accessed through your heart. It is essential that you bring your attention inward.

The first step is to change your relationship with the ego mind and the heart.

The muscle of the heart is very small because you have not been connecting to it. Let's look at how you are going to begin to open up to your heart, expanding your heart muscle.

First, become aware of your physical heart. You need to begin spending time just holding your heart with the palm of the hand, and taking a breath. Bring your consciousness to the feeling of the pressure of the hand and the warmth of the hand on your physical body. By consciousness I mean your awareness, so that all of your attention comes to the physical experience of the pressure of the hand, in this moment. Nothing else—focus only on feeling your hand on your chest. In this very moment you take a breath. This action is powerful. You are being with *your heart,* in the present moment.

I want you to understand the power of being in the moment. We spend our lives thinking of what is to come, or what has happened in the past. We are seldom in the present moment. All we have—all that is truly real—is this moment. When we choose to consciously be in this moment, we connect to our power; we connect to an alignment with Self; we move out of separation. We connect to the clarity of Truth.

It is the ego mind that takes us away from the experience of the moment, constantly worrying about the past or the future. The heart opens us up only into this moment now, and when we connect into the heart and breathe, the breath expands our experience of the moment, our connection to our heart, to our light.

This is how it begins:

Step 1. Bring your hand to your physical heart.

Step 2. Bring your consciousness to the pressure of your hand on your chest.

Step 3. Take a breath; open up to *This is MY heart.* Take a breath.

This Is My Heart

Open up to the need of this heart—*your* heart. It needs a soft breath, a deep breath in through the mouth and just releasing the breath without controlling the out breath. Let the heart open by releasing energy with this breath. You may even release a sigh or sound with the out breath. This is called the Conscious Breath.

Your heart has been waiting for you, for this connection and awakening. Claim your heart; claim yourself with each breath. Most important, claim this moment—your moment with the breath.

Your heart needs resurrecting. It's the time for your heart to come into a self-realization process. This can only happen when you consciously claim your heart. Your heart will transform; you will transform. Yes, YOU!

Be aware that the ego mind has been committed to trying to keep you safe all this time, and now its job needs to change. You have been living in survival up to this point and now it is the time to move into living. All true living is done through the heart.

The ego still has a job to do, but its purpose is to assist you in organizing things in your life, reading tasks, and generally keeping the third-dimensional things in order. That is all you need your ego mind for: to do tasks, not to run your life. The ego is going to have to readjust to its new position, and you are going to need to be loving, patient, and compassionate with the ego mind while the it moves through this transition.

Every time your ego is worrying or afraid, trying to work things out, or being very dramatic and anxious, just bring your hand down onto your physical heart, bring your consciousness to where your hand is holding your heart and begin to take deep, slow Conscious Breaths. Bring all of your consciousness and attention to the heart. You will experience a change in the feelings you are having. You will feel calmer and less agitated. The drama of the feeling will fade away because drama does not exist within the heart. There will be a feeling that things will be all right somehow. You may even experience a solution to the problem at hand, something you were not expected to have thought of yourself—a simple solution.

As you begin to connect through the heart, you connect to the unlimited source of Universal knowledge and understanding, which is a natural link to the light of the Self. This is a natural part of you, a part that you have always had. Now it is time for you to link into this aspect of yourself and utilize the assistance that is here for you.

As you work more with the heart and develop this alignment to the Self, your guidance and connection to the heart will grow and flourish, and you will live more and more in the moment, effortlessly, in the flow of the light of the Self. The heart will become more self-realized, and by this I mean it will begin to do its job the way it was always meant to do.

The words *Thy Will Be Done* reflect the truth of this state. Through your heart you move toward the alignment to the light of the Self, you surrender to your journey, and allow the light of the Self to take you where you need to go, doing what you need to do. Each time you speak these words, *Thy Will Be Done,* you align yourself more and more to light of Self, and anchor yourself in the natural flow and current of that river of light. You let go and allow yourself to flow with *your* life and your journey. It is effortless as you move into that natural flow—that current of your light.

◇◇◇◇◇◇◇◇◇◇◇◇

It is now time to listen the first track (found at *www.christineday-online.com/piol/* and unlocked with code included on card at back of book), called "Transforming the Heart." You will need to listen to this a number of times. Each time you will experience it differently because the audio file holds unlimited energetic levels, and as you are ready it will take you into those deeper initiations. It will take you where you need to go, continuing to expand your heart connection, awakening your heart. There is a language that is channeled through this audio file; this language is from the Pleiadians. It is designed to speak to the light of the Self, the sole essence of you, and to bring your light forward. It is going to help your heart to begin to transform and awaken. It will work within the cells of the heart, healing your heart cells and activating a new life force through the cells as the healing takes place. The heart's cells will begin to respond to the words like a flower opening up to the sun. Each cell in your heart will go through a transformational awakening. Physical healing can take place in your heart as this awakening takes place. Just open up to it and let go; allow it to awaken you. Allow any emotional feelings to just flow out.

As you open to the language that is channeled through you may feel as though you recognize this language on some level: It may feel familiar; it may feel comforting. It carries with it frequencies of love and energies of awakening. Whatever your experience, just breathe and open up to receive this energy within the cells of your heart.

You will transform;

Your heart will transform;

Your life will transform.

It is a time to celebrate you in the moment through your heart. Remember: This is a step-by-step process: one breath at a time, one moment at a time. The spiritual forces will be supporting you during this journey, and I will be with you energetically. The Pleiadians will be present, if you wish to be assisted with them. We open to the Angels, Light Beings, Masters, to witness you and the birth of your heart, the birth of you. We celebrate you as you take this next step.

Have a good journey!

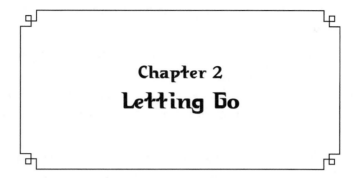

Chapter 2
Letting Go

You have been on this earth plane for many lifetimes, and over a long period of time you have held on to many experiences, many concepts and ideas, and socially expected behaviors that have kept you controlled. This has taken away your personal power. You, of course, have given away your power. No one can ever *take* *it* from you, but in order to be loved or accepted in social settings or family dynamics you conformed to what was expected of you, and bit by bit you gave yourself away.

As children we all quickly learn to do what we need to do in order to survive. We need love, and approval equals love. Children are totally dependent on their caretakers for protection, for food, and just to be taken care of. As I mentioned earlier, we continue to live this way long after we are children. We take this learned behavior into our adulthood and continue to play it out in all our relationships.

There comes a time when we need to acknowledge our behavior as adults and begin to change our behavior. We have to begin to honor ourselves, to love ourselves, and to be patient and gentle with ourselves. We need to be loving, patient, and compassionate toward ourselves as we heal. It takes great courage to decide to do things differently, because there is safety in familiar patterns no matter how painful they are. It's what we know!

Begin by knowing you have a right to be loved and supported in your life. It's time for you to let go and allow yourself to accept that you are really okay. You! Yes, you—just as you are, in this moment. There is nothing you need to change about yourself to receive this love. You have a right to be loved and supported, *now*.

The truth is that the love and support are here for you right in this moment. You only need to reach out to access the love and the help that is here for you. There is an incredible amount of support here for you in this moment and you really don't have to do anything alone again. The struggle can stop, *now*.

It is a part of your natural birthright to have abundance on all levels. You are an important part of the divine plan and you matter. This is a truth. *You matter!*

I want you to take a breath, in the mouth and out the mouth, right now, and let go. Breathe and let go.

You have been holding on for so long, you don't even realize how much you don't breathe. And as you hold everything in, the energy of your feelings goes into the cells of your body; the tension, the pain, and the fear go into your cells. So the cells in your body begin to carry this energy of pain of fear and tension, and with each situation in your life this energy builds up in the cells of your body. Some of this process is about letting go of the buildup in your cells, to free yourself from the pain and the fear. Allow the cells to be free from this burden that you carry; allow yourself to be free!

Take another deep breath in the mouth, and then let the breath out through the mouth. All the tension in the cells begins releasing. This breath in and out of the mouth releases the buildup of stress that goes into the cells. If a sound wants to come out with the breath, let it come;

it's part of the letting go. Sometimes emotion may want to come out with this breath, and that's okay. Let it come. It's time. It's good to *feel* and to *let go.*

As you breathe and the cells begin to let go of the tension of the past, a new aspect of yourself can begin to be birthed. You can begin connecting to some other part of your Self. This type of breath says, "Yes, I am willing to let go. Yes, I am willing to begin to receive my light, and to connect to my light."

Every time you breathe this way another level of you will let go, so you breathe and let go, breathe and let go. Remember: This is called a Conscious Breath. This is you beginning to consciously choose change—to choose to birth yourself. Each breath says, "I open to this birthright now." With each breath you are activating this process of change for yourself. Just let go with the breath, and open up to receiving what is naturally yours.

It reminds me of my journey moving from death back into being alive. With each Conscious Breath I chose life. I chose to liberate myself. So breathe; you choose life: With breath, you choose love. The Conscious Breath is a loving action that you bring to yourself in each moment. You can do this. You have a right to be alive, to be loved, and to be free of the many burdens you carry with you.

Reading these words right now can bring emotional feelings. Many of you have been alone for so long, looking for something that makes sense in your life. You have been trying hard to understand with the mind what is it that will bring meaning to your life—trying to understand how life works and how to move away from cycles in your life that just don't take you anywhere.

The pain that comes from being so separate and lost is sometimes intolerable. The feeling of separation is the lack of connection to yourself—the Self. You just want all the struggle, fear, and pain to stop. You have been in this separation for lifetimes, and now we have been given the grace on this planet to move out of this separation, for the veils to lift and truly move into a new level of awakening. You are moving toward *you*; you are moving toward the light of your Self, moment-by-moment, breath by breath, as you choose life and love. The loving element can come back into your life each time and each moment you choose to breathe.

Just take another breath, breathing in through the mouth, and letting go, breathing out of the mouth, choosing life, choosing love.

As you do this, the story of your life will begin to drop away. What I mean is that the story of your life up to this point will lose its importance. You will no longer cling to the past but see it more as something that has brought you to this moment in time, and nothing else. A series of events that took place, that have given you experiences—nothing more—and from here you can let go and move on toward yourself in a new way.

In a series of steps that follow, you are going to begin to have a change. The first question is: *Are you willing to allow the change?* You don't have to know how to go about this; there is no knowledge required—just a desire for the change. You don't even have to know exactly what that change will look like. You don't have to have these answers right now. All you need to know is that you need and want to change what is happening in your life—that you are willing to change. You have an intention to let go and move toward opening to this new level of yourself.

Your higher Self will begin to set in motion a series of events in your life that will create change. You will need to open up and allow these changes, and for this to happen you must have a willingness to let go and trust. You have everything to gain and nothing to lose here. It's time for you.

The "letting go" energy is powerful. It allows for change to take place, because as the letting-go energy is activated within your cells, the old (all that you have been holding on to) moves out, making room for change and for transformation in the cells of your body. As this transformation takes place within the cells, physical healing can take place within the body. The cells density begins to change and this makes the physical healing possible.

The letting-go energy also transmits throughout all levels of your life. It moves like a wave, rippling through all aspects, helping you break down and clear old ineffective stuck patterns. It opens up new doors, and new opportunities where needed. This letting-go energy ripples out to all areas your life, and you begin to receive your natural abundance. It allows for a healing on all levels: healing in relationships, healing on the physical level, and healing on the emotional level. It is time for you to allow this for yourself.

One woman came to me for help. She was unhappy in her life; she had a job she was unfulfilled in and a relationship that was no longer working, and she was suffering from a lot of physical back pain.

As I spoke with her I found out she was carrying a lot of guilt around a car accident. This accident had happened 20 years earlier, and a person died in that accident. The accident was not her fault, but she was the driver and she had taken on the full guilt, blaming herself for not being able to do something to prevent the accident. As she talked about her experience and her deep feelings of remorse and self-condemnation, I could feel the dense energy around her issue and how she was holding on to her guilt. Even though she could logically agree she was not responsible for the actual accident, she could not let go of the guilt. She spoke of not deserving anything good for herself, and that she deserved to be punished.

I asked her whether she was willing to work with the letting-go energy, explaining that it was an energy that moved through the energetic field and through the cells of the body, releasing any form of energetic hold. It would first loosen old issues, and then help these issues to move out, changing the energetic vibration of her body and within her world.

She agreed, but wasn't very enthusiastic. I told her it really didn't matter how convinced she was; all that mattered was that she would say yes, and just open up to the experience. So I worked with her opening up the letting-go energy process. She promised to be committed during the actual process, and that was all I needed to be able to activate the process so that she could receive the letting-go energy. She actually had a positive experience during the process, feeling like something had lifted and like she didn't feel so heavy with her burden. She felt a small sense of relief and she was willing to open up to the possibility of change. I gave her a CD with the letting-go process and asked her to listen to it three times during the first week. I told her that she didn't have to do anything but listen to the CD and breathe. We agreed to meet two weeks later.

Two weeks later she walked into the room with a very different energy than the last time that I had seen her. She shared with me that her back pain was a lot better and that she had come to the realization of how much emotional pain she had been carrying around with her. She had come to many understandings within herself, in a natural way, as though some wall had come down. She was able to see and understand events differently, and because of this could let the pain go and move on.

She had been given a promotion in her job, and she could feel that there was something new inside of her: She now had a chance to be happy in her life.

This woman continued to listen to the letting-go CD, and step by step, a lot of change took place in her life. The changes within her led to something more positive in her relationship, and she was able to begin to receive differently, and open up to different, more positive experiences in her life.

This is how the letting-go energy works. The most powerful aspect of it is its ability to loosen the hold of old emotional baggage—the baggage that prevents us from being able to receive and move forward in our lives.

I want you to open up to this picture: You are holding onto a branch of a tree with both hands. You are hanging over a river. There is a gentle current flowing in this river. The letting-go energy is calling you to let go. This means you simply need to open your fingers off the branch that you are holding on to, and fall gently into the river below and be taken into the flow—the current of this river. This is an effortless action of just opening the fingers and letting go. You simply fall into the river that takes you with this gentle current. You are being carried, held, and moved forward. There is nothing for you to do except breathe, rest, and allow your self to be carried. This river is *your* river of light, and the flow that you are in is the flow of the light of yourself that will take you where you need to go in this life. This is *letting it go.* There is no effort to it, just a simple act of opening the fingers off the branch you have been holding on to. You have been gripping it tightly for so long, and now you can simply let go. The effort and energy used to hold on are exhausting you. So just let go and allow the light of the self to assist you, *now.* Know that the letting-go energy that is activated on the CD will assist you to move into your river and assist you in being able to let go on this level.

∞∞∞∞∞∞∞∞∞∞

It is now time for you to open to the second audio track (*www. christinedayonline.com/piol/*), channeled from the Pleadians through me to you. It is designed to activate the letting-go process in and through your cells, and through your life. This energy is here for you. It is an exciting moment—a conscious moment as you take a powerful step toward more of yourself.

As you open up to it during this journey it will help you begin to let go of things you have been holding on to. As you let go and the cells begin to let go, light of the Self can begin to anchor into your body. As this happens you begin to be able to connect more to that flow of light in that river. You will have the opportunity to begin to flow with your river of light and to take your place. This will open you more to the light of Self.

Each time you listen to this second track another level of the letting-go energy can be birthed through your cells. Know that I will energetically be with you. I will hold the space for you, supporting your changes and being a witness to all that you let go of, and the transformation and birth of new light within you and the new energies being activated in your life. If you are willing to open up and allow the Pleadian energies to assist you in the letting-go process, it is such a powerful and exciting experience. Just give your permission, and allow your journey. Open up to the language on the audio track. It will also help you connect into another level of Self.

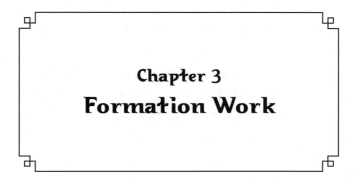

Chapter 3
Formation Work

What Is a Formation?

When you work with a Formation you work with a sacred geometrical form. This sacred form anchors different dimensional spaces for you to open up to the initiation processes that take place within your energetic field and the cells of your body.

The Formation gives you an opportunity to begin to work in dimensional spaces other than the third dimension. It takes you into the fourth-, fifth-, and sixth-dimensional realms where you can work with light aspects of the Self. There is a pure aspect of love that is held within these dimensional spaces, a love that creates transformation and healing within the physical, emotional, and spiritual bodies. This space gives you access and an opportunity to work with an aspect of your higher self and to anchor these light energies of your Self directly into the cells of your physical body. As you access this light of the Self and anchor it into the cells there is an opportunity for physical healing to take place. This light also works within the emotional body. Emotion is held in the cells and as this light comes in the emotional energy can begin to be released. It will open you up to new states of reality as you navigate through the different dimensional states held within the dimensional spaces of the Formation. It will help you accelerate into a deeper connection to your own light Self. You will be initiated by this love.

Each time you work within this energetic vehicle you will unfold more. Each time you decide to work with a Formation journey you will expand and transform energetically. Your cells will expand with your energetic light each time you come back from a Formation journey.

Each journey is unique, and uniquely designed, completely for you. There is a divine orchestration that opens just for you to unfold into, to access teaching of truth and understanding of yourself. As you complete each journey your cells become awakened with your light, you begin to move into a much more conscious state of awareness on an energetic level. The spiritual realms are able to connect with you much more easily as you awaken, as you receive more of your light into your cells. You become even more consciously connected as you birth and initiate into your light Self. Know that you are held in love as you unfold.

The Formation creates a vehicle for you; this vehicle allows you to access and then anchor into energetic alignments to other sacred dimensional spaces. This means that the Formation itself takes you into fourth-, fifth-, and sixth-dimensional openings, where you can heal and transform yourself on many levels. Through the use of sacred geometrical forms, and with the help of the Pleiadians, you will be initiated within these spaces.

Each Formation experience will accelerate you to an alignment with the Universal Consciousness and give you access to an experience of your unique divine aspect of the whole. This means you will begin to open up to direct experiences of your energetic place within the Universe and have a new sense of belonging within a pure loving force. You will experience yourself as a part of that pure loving force. It will move and birth through you, impacting your consciousness and life. It will open up opportunities for you to take your place in the world, and open you up to your natural birthright of unlimited abundance, so you will begin to activate that in your life. With each journey you will birth new levels of your light Self into your cells. Each journey will be different because you will be different. There are an unlimited number of levels for you to anchor into for your initiation, but each journey you take is complete in itself.

Because of the "Self Healing Prophecy," the Pleiadians have given you access to this process because it is now time for us to have this accelerated awakening. My energies can also support you. Part of my gift is an ability to energetically work with each one of you. You only need to call on me energetically and I will be with you. That is my commitment to you. I can hold an energetic platform to assist you in integrating the energy from your journeys in the Formation, so that your cells are fully receiving a new level of your light and that each cell is fully integrated with that light. This is part of my mission here on this earth plane. I am anchored into an unlimited form of myself, and my energies are always available.

How to Get Ready to Do the Formation Work

There are some things you will need to set up in order to be able to do this Formation work. You will need yourself and three other people, OR you will need yourself and three markers, tissues, or cushions. (Note: You do not want to use crystals to mark places.)

The Formation is set up in a perfect square; each of the four positions is marked with either a person or a marker. Depending on the number of people, you use the markers to make up four places. It does not matter how many people or how many markers you have in the formation (as long as the total is four). It is important that you make sure each Formation is aligned correctly, each place being directly opposite the other, or markers lined up so that the square is balanced. You want the spacing between each place to be the same. The actual size of the Formation is unimportant; it can be large or very small, but it must be balanced. The Pleiadians and the Spiritual realms can work much more effectively with you in a properly balanced Formation base. The energies

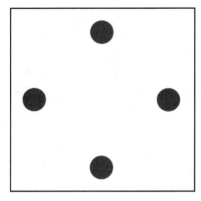

Diagram A

that set up can be much more effective with this properly balanced base. So take your time to make sure that this base is evenly constructed. (See Diagram A.)

The Pleiadians and Spirit can only support the work if these alignments are correct, and you need that support from them. They can assist you with your initiations and your experiences, and especially with the integration of the many levels of light that will be coming into your cells. These energies of your light that you bring back into your body need to be fully utilized, which is achieved by you fully integrating them into the cells. This is where the support of Spirit and the Pleiadians is important. They make sure you are fully integrated as you initiate.

Be aware that the Pleiadians are available to anchor themselves in the spaces of the Formation where there are no people, in the marker positions. They energetically hold those positions to assist you in opening up the sacred geometrical dimensional spaces. So you can work with other people in the Formation, or the Pleiadian energies. The Pleiadians will fill any gaps, so you could have two people and the two marker positions filled by the Pleiadians.

You will need to come into your body before you begin this Formation. That means bringing your energy from your mind down into your body, down especially into your heart. Take the time to connect with your hands on your chest, feeling the pressure and the warmth of your hands. Use the Conscious Breath, in and out of the mouth. This quickly brings you away from your mind and into your body. You cannot be in the Formation experience with the ego mind. The connection into the body is important to do before you begin the Formation meditation, because it opens up the cells of your body in readiness to receive the initiating energy. It consciously opens you up to receive a whole new level of yourself, and it also says to the Universe, "Yes, I am ready!"

Remember that the breath says, " Yes, I am willing to let go"
and "Yes, I am willing to receive." It is important that this be a
conscious act on your part.

My questions to you are: *Are you willing to receive and how much are*
you willing to receive?

It is amazing how little some of us feel we deserve. It is part of our natural birthright to have abundance on all levels. Remember what the Pleiadians ask: "Why have a grain of sand when you can have the whole beach?"

So I hold a space for each one of you to open up and receive all that is your right to receive!

Before you begin, set an intention and specifically open up to receive during this specific Formation, to receive what you are willing to allow. You must ask in order to receive!

Spirit needs to know what it is you desire in order to bring it to you. Be as specific as you can be and then let go, confident and secure in the knowledge that the process for receiving it is under way.

If you are doing the Formation with other people it is good to have others witness your personal intention for your journey. If you are alone, bring your intention forward, and allow the Pleiadians and Spirit to witness your intention.

It is also important to invite support for your journey in the Formation *before* you begin. This can be from the Pleiadians, Spirit, me, or any of your individual alliances. It is my experience that all energies can support here. There is only oneness—no separation.

The Formation is a pure light space. There is no need to feel as though you must protect yourself. Because it is a pure light space there is no possible opening available for any unwanted energies. The Formation holds an incredible space in which you can fully integrate the light that you bring back into your own cells after the completion of the journey. It is similar to a womb creating an enclosed energetic space in which you can rest and integrate. You are held in a loving light space.

In the Beginning

When you first open up to the Formation energy it is important to just *allow* your full experience and not necessarily follow all my directions and words on the third audio track (*www.christinedayonline. com/piol/*). Know that sometimes your experiences will take you away from my voice. This is really okay, and actually very important. It means you are in the flow of your unique experience. It's powerful and you are being totally taken into an aspect of your own healing in that moment. You can totally trust this when it happens; just go with what is happening to you. Trust and allow.

At other times you may feel extremely sleepy. This happens when there is a high level of new light being integrated into the cells. This means you are aligning with new dimensional aspects of yourself. These are higher states of your light anchoring through you, so the cells integration of this expanded energy creates a sleepy state. Just let go and allow the process. There may be times that you go into a sleep-like state. This is not sleep, but you are being moved into another dimensional space for a deeper healing process. This often takes place when there is a significant process of healing going on within your energetic field.

There may be times when you don't remember anything of the journey. This happens when there has been a deep energetic alignment to the Self. You are completely taken out of the way—which means the ego mind cannot interfere with this important step—while this process is happening. When you come back from a journey like this, it is important to take a lot of time to breathe and integrate the energy into the cells of your body. This light energy that you have brought back with you is a new level of your own light self, healing energy that can transform your cells and transform your energetic field.

It is important not to try to visualize any part of your experience. By visualize I mean don't try to see something. If something comes to you naturally and you see it, perfect. But the *trying* is the ego mind wanting to interfere, the ego mind wanting to play a part, and wanting to control, and the ego mind will stop your experience ultimately. Understand that the ego mind will not be able to operate within these fourth/fifth- and sixth-dimensional levels. It cannot function there. So if you are in your ego mind your true experiences will happen energetically, but you will not be able to have a direct experience of them as they are happening.

If you find yourself in your ego mind and you are not having any experiences, you need to simply put your hand on your heart and breathe, bringing your consciousness into your hand and into your heart. This will bring your energy back into your body and away from the ego mind. It's a simple process. At the beginning you may find your mind interfering; that's okay. Be patient and loving to the ego, and simply bring yourself gently back into your body and resume your journey.

Simply open up to what is happening in each moment; just be with each experience by bringing your consciousness to it, and taking a breath. This is being in the moment. The more you bring your consciousness to each experience and breathe, the more expansion of that particular experience will take place in that moment.

Some of your experiences may be subtle; open up to the subtle energy that is there, and let yourself be with it. You and the energy: letting go and breathing; being in the moment. Let yourself unfold into it. When you are willing to be with what is right in front of you and open to that, whatever the experience, your experience opens and expands more. The more you are willing to open up to that experience, the more you will be moved and opened into deeper experiences.

Be aware that the Formation space is a fourth/fifth- and sixth-dimensional space, so you are going to find yourself having very different experiences than this third-dimensional earth plane. There is of course no time—no fixed boundaries—and you may experience yourself very differently as you open into new energetic aspects of yourself. The mind will not understand any of your experiences; it is outside the realm of your mind. It is through your heart and the cells of your body that truth from the higher levels is recognized and understood. Through the formation energies you will receive a new level of clarity, understanding, and information that you need for your next steps in your life.

Once you and your three other positions are set up you can begin to open to the third audio track, which will begin the activation of your Formation journey.

Anchoring the Base

The first step is to anchor the Base of your Formation. Be sure that you are *in your body,* remembering that you need to be aligned with the body. Use your breath to do this. You want to *consciously* take your place in the base of the Formation, claiming your place here, anchoring yourself like roots of a tree. Feel those roots going down into the earth. As you do this you will begin to experience your place more completely within the Formation Base. Let yourself open up fully to your place here in the Base. It is powerful to truly feel being here, taking your place and willing to show up for yourself in this moment.

You are going to create a Base of your Formation. The first step is for you to bring your consciousness or focus to the person on your left. As you do so, an energetic line is going to form between you and the person on your left, or the Pleiadian energy on your left. (See Diagram B.) Know that, wherever you bring your attention or consciousness, an energetic line is created. This is a universal truth, so as you do this in the formation it creates a connection.

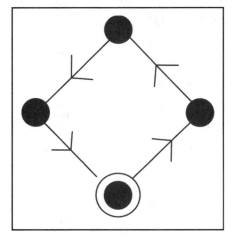

Diagram B

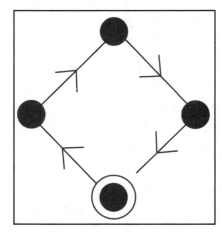

Diagram C

As everyone within your Formation does this, there is a line created connecting each one of the four positions in the Formation, and the Base is birthed. (See Diagram C on page 84.)

The Base, as it births, opens up the first energies of another dimensional space. Bring yourself deeper into your place within the Base as it opens. Breathe and anchor yourself more. You will—on some level—experience a changing state (occurring where you are). Let go and allow yourself to expand with it. Know that the change may be subtle; it may be strong; it does not matter. Just bring your consciousness into the Base in that moment and breathe.

You will then bring your consciousness or attention to the person on your right, and as you do so an energetic line will form between you and the person on your right. Doing this expands and strengthens the Base, bringing even more changing energies as the Base opens up even further, and your experience of the Base expands even more. You may experience a union between you and the Base, almost as though you have somehow become part of the base. It may seem as though the Base is much larger, or smaller, or maybe tilted in some way. It may feel as though the Base is fluid. It does not need to make sense on a third-dimensional level. Remember: This is not a third-dimensional space you are entering; it is a fourth-, fifth-, and sixth-dimensional space.

You may feel and experience yourself very differently here; you are different. You are accessing different energetic aspects of yourself as you open into a new dimensional realm!

Then bring your focus and connect with the person opposite you. As you open to this connection there is a stronger energetic line that forms. (See Diagram D at right.)

As you bring a deeper focus to that connection and take a breath, this energetic line expands and grows

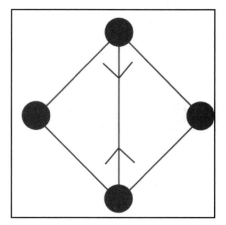

Diagram D

stronger. The connecting line opposite of you deepens, strengthens, and opens in some way as you bring more of your attention to this connection.

As you are connected into the Base and are part of the Base, you change and expand. New energies of light begin to birth through your cells. It may feel as though you and the Base are somehow merging. It can be that you begin to experience the Base getting larger and larger, filling the whole room. Or you may experience it very differently. It does not matter what your experience is; the important thing is that you just keep opening up to your experience, bringing your full consciousness to whatever your experience is, allowing it, letting go, and breathing.

The Apex

The Apex position is generally set above you; however, it sometimes can be to the side of you or even beneath you. It may be either very far away from you or very close. It does not matter which; the important thing to understand is that the Apex is there. You may see it, feel it, or sense it. There is no importance as to *how* you experience it.

The Apex has its own light consciousness. It is an energetic light form. You are going to need to greet the Apex. This means to bring your consciousness up toward this energy in order to greet it. It doesn't matter how

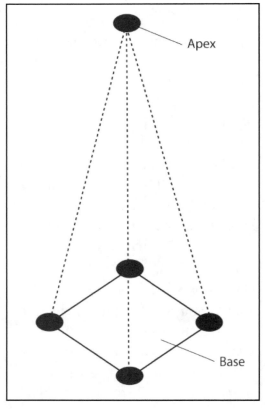

Diagram E

you greet the Apex. It may be just acknowledging its presence like a stranger on the street, saying hi. Or you may have the experience of meeting a beloved dear friend that you have not seen for a long time—deeply loving—and you experience a strong connection through your heart. As you do this, the Apex will respond by sending its own light connection down toward you, and down into the Base.

Remember the rule: Wherever your consciousness goes, an energetic line forms. So as you bring your consciousness to the Apex, a line of energy is formed. (See Diagram E.)

As the Apex sends its energy down to each marker position, an energetic line forms from above down into the Base, creating a Sacred Pyramid form. (See Diagram E.) This form begins to anchor into the Base, anchoring through you. As the Pyramid anchors its energy into the Base of the Formation, the Base begins to transform on another level. It opens up, and as it does you need to bring your connection deeper into the Base. It may feel like you *are* the Base; this is okay. Move with your experiences!

The Pyramid

The energy of the Sacred Pyramid is unlimited in form and its multi-dimensionality. This sacred form allows for an unlimited amount of experiences to take place for you within the sacred structure, and there are an unlimited number of initiating processes waiting for you as you are ready to unfold. Each initiating experience is monitored and supported by the Pleiadians and the Spiritual forces.

When I talk about your experience being monitored I mean that the Pleiadians will make sure that the light energies you take in will not be too much for your electrical system to integrate, and you will be constantly supported in your ability to integrate these energies.

There will be new experiences opening up for you every time you work with its sacred energies. The Pyramid has a series of initiation energies that will take you deeper and deeper into yourself. Let go and allow this sacred energy to work within you; let go and let your journey unfold. The more relaxed you are, the more you will be able to receive the channeled guidance that is available to you within the Formation. The more you allow your own experience, the more you will be able to open to these new levels of yourself within the different dimensional spaces.

Your cells will go through a rapid energetic change, and the Formation energy will assist you in fully integrating these energies.

The Column of Light

Once the Pyramid is anchored into the Base there is a Column of Light that comes down from the Apex, down into the base of the Formation. The Column of Light is also a separate consciousness; its function is different from the Apex. (See Diagram F at left.) The Column holds a powerful quality of love and can be accessed by bringing your consciousness toward its light. The Column's light gives you a direct opening into the higher aspect of your light Self. It is a teacher, bringing you knowledge and awakening. It helps you open up your consciousness so that you can more readily be aware of the energies that are here to assist you in your journey on this earth plane. It is important to breathe when you open up to the Column's energy. As you work with these energies they will help you open up much more completely to the expanded light energy of the Column, and integrate this energy into your cells of your body.

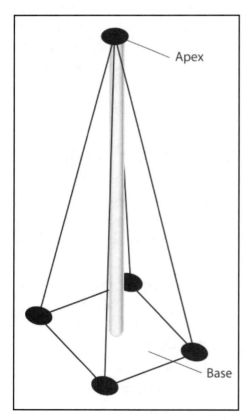

Apex

Base

Diagram F

The Column brings a healing energy and light to the cells of your body, which opens a flowing access to the Self. It gives you access, like a teacher, for you to open and receive new understandings and information about your own path and journey. The more you are willing to let go, the more the Column of Light can work with you. The Column will open up new channeling alignments. These channeling alignments will begin to build and expand through you, giving you access to direct communication from the Self and the Spiritual realms. As your own channel becomes more defined within you, it allows you to access a deeper level of communication with the Spiritual realms, and to the energies and alignment to the Self. The communication with the Self brings you clarity of your path and journey, as well as the steps that need to be taken to move you in the direction you need to go. It brings you an understanding of your journey and a new level of clarity with which to work within your day-to-day living here on this earth plane.

This understanding and clarity make it much easier to navigate your way through the third-dimensional illusion—to move and flow in the higher dimensional experiences on a daily basis. They allow you to be conscious in the day-to-day living in this third-dimensional world and assist you in navigating through your life in a conscious way, moment by moment, so you are able to stay consciously aligned during your experiences here. This is how you move into this energetic flow of your own light. These initiations will give you this access to clarity. With the clarity you connect to your own personal power and move naturally to co-create your world.

In the Formation, many times the Column fills the Pyramid space with its consciousness, and as it does so the Pyramid energy expands its energy into other dimensional levels of itself. It can also move down through your physical body. It works within your cells and, as it creates these new channeling alignments, creating new connections for you to work with, it adjusts your energetic levels to allow you to expand your energies more completely. You will find that you develop your own individual relationship with the consciousness of the Column. Communication with the

Column happens as you bring your consciousness toward the Column. It can begin to communicate with you through a thought-transference process. This energetic way of communicating can bring to you knowledge and assist you in an understanding of truth and alignments for your Self. As this communication takes place you are able to develop a relationship and deeper connection to the Column and to this consciousness of light. It is up to you whether you choose to develop this relationship or not.

Sacred Spiral Energy

The Sacred Spiral's energy is found in the Column of Light. (See Diagram G.) It moves down through the Column, into the Pyramid, and into you. The Spiral's major role is to integrate the energies of light through your cells. It also breaks down the barriers of the ego, allowing you to more easily access the energy of the heart. It gives you support in traveling through the dimensional spaces as they open up. The Spiral has a separate consciousness. When the Spiral is present, you will often experience a physical movement through your body. It can be a very deep physical experience. Trust this and just let go as the spiral takes you energetically where you need to go. Allow your own transformation to take place as the Spiral unravels you with its energy and movement. This

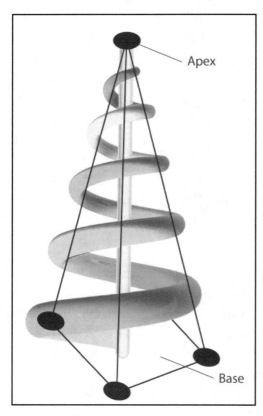

Diagram G

unraveling is important because you are like a tight ball letting go. The Spiral opens you up so that you can receive the light, and heal through the cells, releasing the "holding on," the struggle and the tiredness in the cells.

You are going to be building sacred relationships with the Apex, Pyramid, Column of Light, and Sacred Spiral. These relationships will have a lasting and powerful impact on you, supporting you in your transformation on an ongoing daily basis. You can truly relax and allow a natural alliance to take place, because this is a natural process. These conscious energies are here to support you in your different stages of birth. There are many levels to the birth of you: you birthing you with the support and love of Spirit, and the Pleiadians. These energetic forces are here to help; they have always been here to help. Open up to receive the abundance that is your natural birthright to receive. Open up to the many levels of help available to you *now*. Be willing to receive.

Remember that each person will take his or her place differently in the Formation; one is not more than the other. So if you are with other people doing this Formation, you will each have a unique individual experience. It's important to understand that you are not dependent on anyone within the Formation for your individual experience. Your experience is completely up to you and what help you will allow during the Formation.

There will be times during these Formation journeys that you may be given information, teachings, energetic symbols, and forms. These energetic tools are initiating energies that you are ready to receive. They may be just for you, or they may be for you to share in the world, but you can trust what you receive. Open your heart wide and receive the gifts as they are given to you. Know that they are given with great love.

These gifts are only given when you are ready to receive them and ready energetically to use them. It is essential to bring your consciousness toward these energies that come in the form of symbols, and to take a Conscious Breath. This will help the cells in your body to be able to integrate and utilize these energies more completely. What you are actually doing is reclaiming aspects of your personal power and integrating them into your energetic field.

Troubleshooting

If you are having problems not experiencing anything in the formation:

1. The most common issue is that you are not coming fully into your body. Most of your energy is in the ego mind, so you are missing out on your experience. You need to place your hands on your chest, feel the pressure of your hands on your chest, and take a breath. As you do so your energy will come away from your ego mind and you will come into the body. This can be done before starting the Formation or during the Formation.

2. You are trying to visualize your experience, which means your mind is trying to make something happen or to see something. This will stop your experience because the mind cannot connect to the true energies of these dimensional spaces. The mind is limited in what it can connect to. So as above, come into your body and away from your ego mind. You need to "actively wait" for something to happen. This means just relax while you wait and breathe until you begin to either see or sense or feel something happening. Then bring your attention to that experience and take a breath.

3. Sometimes in the Formation you may experience one aspect of the Formation more strongly than another. For example, the Base may be very subtle, almost non-existent, and the Apex or Pyramid may be very strong. Sometimes you need a stronger energetic of one consciousness more than another for your unfolding, so in this situation you will experience one form of the Formation more than the other. You can trust it. Your needs vary from journey to journey.

Allow yourself to move your body as you need to. Your body may need this movement to integrate the new energy entering the cells of your body. The movement opens the cells to your initiating light, allowing the transformation. And sometimes with this movement of light in the cells, there is a sound that needs to be released from you. It may be like a loud sigh, or it can be a very loud sound or tone. This is dense energy leaving the body. These dense energies can sometimes leave through sound. It allows a deep healing to take place in that moment; this is freedom for you.

Be aware that sometimes the sounds can act as integrators, and sometimes they can align you to your personal power. Don't hold back your sound; it is powerful. Allow yourself to become the sound and let go into the sound.

After your Formation process it is helpful and supportive to lie down and give yourself plenty of time to integrate all that you have received. Often during this time you realize how much you have received on your journey. You begin to open to the healing energy moving through your body, and to the received insights and information that you need for your next step in your journey. Breathe into your body and let go, opening to receive.

◊◊◊◊◊◊◊◊◊◊◊◊◊

It is now time to listen to the third audio track. I will energetically be with you in this process. Open up to the support of the Pleiadians, Spirit, and any energies that you individually work with to assist you in this journey. Have fun! Breathe and be alive!

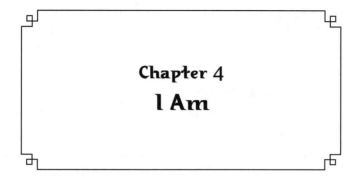

Chapter 4
I Am

The most powerful statement you can make are the words *I am.* These simple words, spoken consciously, activate a truth. These words make a statement to the Universe of you owning your unique divine place within the oneness, and consciously claiming your place. This is tremendously powerful. It starts a wave of reaction throughout the Universe, activating your energetic signature wave outward. You begin to be aligned within the Universe through your cells with this energetic light wave as it creates an energetic opening. Each one of us has a unique place on the Universal grid within the Universal Consciousness.

I liken it to a jigsaw puzzle. Your unique piece can only fit within this place. So as you claim your place with the words *I am,* you activate your energy within your place on the Universal grid. It vibrates and expands in light each time you acknowledge it, using the words *I am.* It goes out into the Universe, and your unique signature of light radiates out, creating a brilliant wave of your light across the Universe, anchoring on this earth plane within your life. This activation of your alignment also creates an awakening in your cells, so that each cell begins to align with your place on the Universal grid. As you speak the words *I am* you are increasingly anchoring your place into the Universal Consciousness within your place on the grid. Every cell vibrates with this activated divine essence, which creates a new level of quickening within the cell. This quickening is a new life force energy that comes from the activation of your place within the Universal grid. With this alignment, healing begins to take place within your physical body.

This Self-Realization process is you beginning to align with your energetic blueprint for this lifetime—the blueprint you chose for yourself. It's what you decided to achieve here: your mission and your lessons. So the awakening to your blueprint is you consciously aligning to the energy of your blueprint, and then beginning to consciously and actively live it in your life. Each time you use the words *I am,* it aligns you into another level of this blueprint. It activates another level of the divine aspect of you, bringing this essence of Self into your life in a powerful way. It is you birthing you with the words *I am.*

You are being called now to begin this powerful activation within yourself. It is the time for you to take your place within the whole. You are needed *now.* You are being called to step forward, consciously, and take your place within the Universe, using the words *I am.* There is a huge difference when you take a conscious step forward—the moment you take your power back and say, "Yes, I am here! I claim my place; I have a place. *I am!*"

Every cell in your body begins to respond—to quicken and align to your energetic flow of your place within the Universe. You experience your place opening up on this earth plane, and you move into a new sense of flow within your life. Your cells begin to vibrate in a new way because they become more alive as they align with this energy of your Self and create a new alignment to all life forms throughout the entire universe. It opens you up the direct experience of a union to all things; you begin to experience a new sense of oneness, and an incredible love that actually begins birthing through your cells. You begin to vibrate love!

As you begin to open to that vibration of love, you recognize and remember that this love exists in everything, in every moment. The truth is that you are love. We are asking you to open up to the miracle of yourself, and embrace *you.*

As you say the words *I am,* feel the power within you; feel how the cells begin to vibrate and align. Use your breath as you speak the words; the breath assists in this alignment. Be aware of your heart, placing your hand on your heart and bringing your consciousness to it. The love is activated through the cells of your heart. A heart awakening takes place. It can be an emotional moment as joy begins to transform the heart.

What a challenge to live consciously and be a catalyst for the world! Each time we meet a part of ourselves and unfold into that part of us, we break through for others to also heal, transform, and to begin to connect, so that they can take their place within the universal whole. Be aware that this is a remembrance process. You are waking up and taking your power back, re-aligning yourself, and re-aligning the cells so you begin to vibrate with the fourth/fifth/sixth-dimensional energies.

Now that you are beginning to live in alignment to your heart, with the new vibration of love (*I am*), it is time to open up to a new way of being and living in the world. When you are living in a conscious state, open to what is around you, you begin to take responsibility for what is happening in your world. This makes it possible to then open up to the messages and gifts that are present for you, and be able to utilize these gifts. Actually you become the gift for the world, being all that you can be in each moment. As you activate your unique energetic signature of you on the Universal grid, it is truly the beginning of your self-realization process.

How we choose to live, the discipline that we have, and the devotion we have to ourselves, dictate what our experiences are going to be. Self-devotion is a key component to your continual unfolding of Self, and part of that devotion is to set a discipline within yourself. This creates a self-loving action that opens our hearts to joy. So what we do and how we do things in our world have a direct result on the experiences we create for ourselves. How we meet or greet those experiences or challenges in each moment, and the actions we take, are what create our world. We live the result of our actions. It's like planting seeds in a garden; we reap what we sow.

There is no separation in this universe: As you give to yourself, others automatically receive. We are not separate from anything; there is only oneness. This is a Truth. As you meet the *I am* energy in your world, there will an expansion of yourself that takes place, and in that expansion you will feel a greater awareness of this light aspect of you. It will feel as though you have somehow become more defined to yourself. There will be a deeper sense of belonging, because of the unity aspect of the *I am* energy. You will automatically be more focused on yourself in each moment, which will allow you to automatically be present for everyone else. You will become a natural healing force in this universe because you are connected into the oneness. When we live in that place we are automatically aligned with others. It is part of the divine economy of life; we connect to the God essence of others as part of the universal whole, and that allows us to naturally hold a space for each person to birth him/herself into their light, and to claim his or her birthright, when he or she is ready.

Each person chooses his or her moment to align with the Self; it is not our responsibility when he or she chooses to do so. It's important to honor each person's individual process, and the way he or she chooses to live in each moment. But it is amazing how powerful it can be for others to witness your unfolding. It is through your living example that others can become inspired to take their steps. The energy you carry as you move through the world impacts all who come in contact with you. When we put our attention on someone else, we leave ourselves and we leave the moment, and when you leave the moment you go into separation. We tend to put our attention on someone else when we don't want to feel what is going on inside ourselves.

Everything that we do creates a reaction in the world: every action and every thought. Thoughts and actions create a wave of energy that goes out into the world, so you can make a difference on this earth plane. We can consciously create each moment when we connect to the *I am.* Part of the third-dimensional illusion is the feeling that we can't possibly be that powerful, and that we don't make a difference in this universe. In actuality we are so powerful with our thoughts that each one of us has an opportunity in each moment to co-create here on the earth plane and within the whole universe!

We can walk gently on this earth plane, gently but powerfully taking our place and moving with a consciousness, love, and respect for all life, including ourselves!

Life Is the Teacher

Each moment of life is a gift. We are being asked to consciously work with what comes to us in our lives consciously. We are not victims; we are given choices every moment of how we respond to each situation in our lives. Each response actually comes down to two reactions: love or fear. The key is to recognize the messages that are held in each life situation presented to you, and then to understand what experiences brought you to that moment. Learn how to internalize and work with the feelings that are present from your experience. There is a simple process to this. The feelings are key, so the question to ask yourself is: *"What am I feeling now?"*

When you can get to the *feeling,* and allow yourself to be with the feeling, your fear response can change to a sense of peace and clarity. *Feeling* is to set yourself free because, once you feel what is there, the energy around your situation transforms.

Many of us are afraid of our feelings. Know that your feelings are not who you are; feelings cannot hurt you. Give yourself permission to just feel. You do not have to justify what the feeling is; it doesn't have to make sense and it doesn't have to be logical to your ego mind. Just allow yourself to be with that feeling as completely as you can, and then it can leave your body. As you do this you will begin to experience a sense of freedom, a deep relief, and a dropping away of something inside of you. The more you are willing to feel in the moment, the more you will be able to move and flow with life, and you will have a new clarity.

When you consciously embrace this truth that life is the teacher, you gain your freedom. You gain it because you no longer believe you are the victim. Instead, you take an active and responsible role in your life. You begin to meet life's experiences in a conscious way.

Life is like an ocean: The waves never stop coming. Some are small and playful, some are huge and come crashing down, but the waves never stop coming. So it is with life; there is the constant movement and challenge in life, and it never stops. The only thing you can count on is that the sun will rise each day, and the days and situations continue to come. You cannot control the situations that arise, and you cannot control what other people will do. But you can count on yourself, and the way you choose to meet each experience. You can open up to yourself, and anchor into the *I am.*

You can walk toward the waves with your heart open, and when the wave comes you can let it pick you up, and place you back down on your feet.

You can walk toward the wave and dive under it.

Or you can let the wave come crashing down on top of you.

As you begin to live more and more in your heart, with the *I am* energy, you will begin to experience a big difference in how you meet the waves in your life. You will have a new clarity about the situations in your life, and this understanding will make it much easier for you to deal with the solutions.

The light of the Self will be able to open you up to creative solutions. You will begin to work with this clarity in your day-to-day life. Your alignment to the love that is activated by the *I am* will take you deeper and deeper into the truth and clarity of the Self, bringing you to a self-realized state of living.

Now I want you to open up consciously to this alignment with the *I am* energy. Begin by bringing your hands to your chest and taking a breath. Follow the breath in and out, in and out. Consciously let go and bring yourself deeply into your awareness in your body: you breathing you; you feeling you, in this moment—nothing but you and the breath.

I want you to consciously begin to open to the words *I am.* Speak the words. Close your eyes. Breathe. You can speak the words out loud or silently to yourself. *I am.* As you say the words, be conscious of you beginning to claim your place here in the Universe, and as you open up and say *yes* to this, speak the words again: *I am.*

Let go, in this moment. Let go of all things in this third-dimensional world, resting in the truth of the Self, as you open up saying the words again: *I am.* You may feel a deep peace as you open up to the energy that is activating through you, as this new alignment begins to be activated in your cells. It might be subtle; it might be strong. There may be a deep sense of relief as this connection is being made. Remember, you are taking back your power, opening up to your place. With each statement of I AM the alignment grows. You can speak the words throughout your day, building the alignment, through your cells and through the heart.

Know that I am energetically with you on your journey. I welcome you as you take this next step forward. There is celebration as you consciously take your place within the Universal Consciousness. There is a strong quickening with your place on the Universal grid as you activate this alignment within the cells of your body.

◇◇◇◇◇◇◇◇◇◇◇◇

Now listen to the fourth audio track (*www.christinedayonline.com/ piol/*). Each time you listen to it you will open to new alignments of yourself. It has been designed for your birth. Let go and allow your own experiences to unfold each time you listen to the CD. Open to your support system that is in place for all of your journeys here. Remember that you can call in help from Spirit and the Pleiadians if you want them. The Pleiadians and Spirit are with you, witnessing your birth and celebrating you!

Have a great journey!

Chapter 5
Thy Will Be Done

W hat do the words *Thy Will Be Done* mean? It is a powerful statement of letting go, surrendering to your divine aspect of your Self, allowing yourself to be guided by that Self, and bringing the ego mind back into its original role of working with organizing the third-dimensional tasks of your life.

Surrendering to the Divine Self allows the light of yourself to guide you through life, opening up to trusting this guidance and moving with this guidance. It is a statement of you activating this connection and saying *"Yes, I open up and allow myself to be shown the way and commit to following my guidance through my sacred heart by the light of my Self."*

So as you make the statement "Thy Will Be Done," you anchor into a flow of light, which is the flow of your unique divinity. Your alignment to this will move you in a new direction in your life. This energetic flow will take you in the direction of living that aligns you to your unique mission that you have come here to experience and complete in this lifetime. The flow will move you into new levels of experience that will awaken you into the energetic flow of your Self. This awakening will activate a deeper conscious connection to this aspect of Self. You will sense the effortless experience of living in the flow of your light. As this connection to the flow deepens, you will experience yourself in a new way. Trust is an important ingredient in the beginning steps of this process. When you first open to this alignment of the flow, you do not allow the ego mind to sabotage your first steps. Trust allows doors of new opportunity to open, and when these doors open you simply take a breath, trust, and walk through that doorway into something new. There is a new sense of truth that begins to vibrate through you as you take these steps.

If you simply hold your heart and breathe you will be able to feel your heart respond to the truth, and the next step that you are about to take will expand its energy. This means you will feel the next step more completely. When in doubt always hold the heart, and bring your consciousness to the heart and breathe. The idea will get stronger if it's part of the flow, or weaker if it is from the ego mind. This process always works, and it will help you in the beginning stages of this changing journey you are on, as you adjust to this new way of being and gain confidence in this new way of living.

Each time you speak the words *Thy Will Be Done*, the alignment strengthens and expands through you, actually linking you deeper into the flow of Self. This truth is calling forward the "light of the Self." Just go with the current of your light, like the current in a river, effortlessly allowing yourself to be taken on your path and held by the light of the Self.

These words do not give away your power; they take you toward aligning more completely to your power. You are simply opening up to a higher dimensional aspect of yourself, your light Self, each time you align with the statement "Thy Will Be Done." You have always had the ability to access this aspect of yourself, even though up to this point you have needed to be in the third-dimensional human being experience of separation.

Now is the time for your awakening, and it's important for you to do so consciously: consciously showing up for yourself; taking conscious action; and claiming the Divine aspect of you. Not only claiming it, but aligning consciously with yourself in this new way.

You are actually aligning with your flow. This flow is an energetic light of the Self that can assist you in your life to move in a direction of abundance on all levels. This is your natural abundance, part of your natural birthright that each one of us has a divine right to receive. Each one of us has our own abundance. It's impossible to have too much, or to take any one else's, so you can freely open to it all, knowing that everyone has access to their own abundance when they are ready to receive it.

Flow

What does this mean, *flow*? The flow is your energetic alignment to a current. You are part of this current; it is your own divine unique signature of the whole—the Universal Consciousness or Oneness. Being connected to the flow of this river is to be brought into alignment with your divine aspect of your light, so you align with the natural rhythm and current of the Self. You enter your river and are effortlessly taken by this current, opened up to new pathways that give you an access into an unlimited level of multidimensional energies and aspects of yourself. This allows you to open up into new levels of understanding and clarity within your life, within this world. It is up to you how much you are willing to open up to in each moment; there are unlimited levels of information and energy available to you in every moment of your experience for you to tap into and become a part of. As you move into your part of this flow you experience a new sense of peace and quiet. You will be naturally aligned to where you are supposed to be in your life because the flow takes you into this alignment.

When you are connected to this natural flow you are being carried into a natural state of birthing yourself, so that you can thrive with the energetic support within the universal energy. It allows your cells to align with a new life force of your spiritual self so that healing can take place on all levels. This divine aspect of your light—we will call it the *Self*—is here to assist you in living your mission on this earth plane, supporting you and guiding you into your natural birthright of abundance on all levels.

Each cell begins a resurrection and realignment to the truth, as though there is a whole new awakening taking place. It starts in the cells of the heart. It is as though you begin to resonate on a whole different level with an expanded life force, and as this happens you begin to draw toward you new experiences, new people, and new opportunities. You begin to align with what is rightfully yours within this universe.

Your sense of clarity will lead you where you need to go. The words *Thy Will Be Done* continue to activate this process deeper and deeper, aligning your cells to the truth and clarity of your life.

There is a surrendering that needs to take place—a surrendering of the ego mind to the heart. The heart is directly connected to your Self. So in reality you hand over the ego mind to your heart—to a direct connection to the light of the Self. You hand over the worry, struggle, and fear to the light of the Self, and move into this flow that will move you toward joy, self- fulfillment, and clarity. You will move out of the third-dimensional illusion of struggle, fear, and lack, and align with the fourth-, fifth-, and sixth-dimensional energies that take you into aspects of your unlimited Self. This unlimited Self can create, source from the unlimited love of the universe, and self-heal.

With the alignment of these dimensional spaces you leave behind the feeling of "lack"; you open the prison door that you have put yourself in for lifetimes, resurrect yourself from limitation, and *lack*. You claim yourself in your unlimited potential.

We have been waiting for you to take your place. No one can fill this place that belongs to you.

As a result of constant worry, fear, and struggle, there has been a buildup of stress that holds within your cells. The built-up stress creates a dis-ease state within the body, and from this Disease is created. But when you are in alignment with the flow of your light, this stress and dis-ease that have been held within your cells can begin to leave the body. As stress leaves the cells, the energy of the light of the Self enters the cells, and regeneration takes place through all your organs and cells of the body. Your physical healing begins to take place.

As you let go of the struggle of *trying* and just begin *being*, your energy levels will begin to expand, because you are no longer using up your energy in the "trying." This brings you into a new level of awareness—a sense of freedom and connection to yourself. You will move into this state of Being as you, more and more, let go into the Flow. Your Flow is taking you toward your heart's desire, moving you toward your heart's passion. When you are doing what you are passionate about you become truly alive, and in that aliveness there is a new state of being that gets birthed within you. You live through your heart, and there are love and passion in your existence. You bring that love and passion to the world.

As you are being moved along this river of light, taken by the current, you will become aware that this river is feeding into an ocean of light. This ocean of light is the Collective Consciousness, the Oneness. As you feed into this ocean, it's as though you become even more defined and even more expanded within this energetic state. You do not lose yourself here, but rather become even more defined within your unique divine aspect of this whole energy of the Universe. You flourish. You bring a uniqueness of spirit to this place, and there is a celebration of you. You are fully received for all that you are and all that you bring. There is a quality of love that exists within this space that is uplifting and glorious. We have been waiting for you—waiting for you to take your place here!

You have not come to this earth plane to just settle for something that does not fulfill you. You have a right to joy, and a right to love and fulfillment. The Flow aligns you to a new direction, where there is a passion for the things you do, and a purpose. The light of the *Self* will guide and direct you and the whole universe will support this flow, opening up the doorways of possibility for you.

Your life will undergo level upon level of transformation as you align more, and more. This alignment helps you work within yourself in a new way, being much more productive in the way you approach your day-to-day living. You begin to take much more responsibility for what you draw to yourself in the way of experiences in your life, understanding that challenges bring you a deeper healing within yourself and an understanding of a deeper meaning of life and living. You no longer feel out of control with the events around you, like a victim, but are conscious that you can use these life experiences as growth tools. You can open up to them like a gift in the moment. Your heart will be opened to give you access to your feelings, moment by moment, and you will be truly present with each moment. When this happens you move out of separation with the Self. You have many tools now to work with, to assist you to be in your body, to consciously work with your feelings.

When something is not working in your life it's not that you are being punished.

It's the universe pointing out to you that maybe you should be doing something differently, or there may be something you need to feel in this moment. It is important to examine what is taking place within the situation. Ask yourself, "*What is going on inside that I need to feel?*"

You need to feel so that you can clear what is there, and then you can move on and the situation can flow again. This is the way you can keep connected to the flow, and allow it to continue to move through your life.

Each moment holds a unique quality of love that you can receive. This is neverending and part of our divine gifts here. It can only be experienced through the heart, when you are in the flow. This flow is the gift, your gift to yourself. All solutions are within the flow; all knowledge is within the flow. There is rest for you here.

◇◇◇◇◇◇◇◇◇◇◇◇

When you listen to the fifth audio track (*www.christinedayonline. com/piol/*), I encourage you to give permission to Spirit and the

Pleiadians to work with you so you get the full benefit of the energy that is here for you. It is your time to open to your flow; this is the beginning. Each time you listen to the audio files it will take you into a deeper place within your flow.

Let go, and allow your Self to take you!

Remember to breathe into all the cells in your body, acknowledging each cell. Open to your healing. It is very important not to necessarily follow all of my instructions, but to be with your experience in every moment. Bring your full consciousness to it and take a breath. You may have an experience of being in a sleep-like state, which is a dimensional doorway, a place of high light frequencies beyond this third-dimensional space. It is where healing takes place. If you are having a problem not being able to have an experience, take some time with your hands on your heart, breathing, feeling your body, and being with your breath.

The language from the Pleiadians is important for you to open up to; it will assist you to open more to your flow, and expand into your place more completely within the ocean of light.

After listening to the audio file make sure you drink plenty of water to help the cells integrate this new level of your light and anchor into your cells. This light is higher aspects of your own light.

Have a great journey!

Chapter 6
Forgiveness of the Self, Resurrection of the Self

There are some important internal emotional processes necessary for resolution with other people or yourself, and situations in your life. These processes free you up energetically so that you no longer have internal wars going on, which create a separation within yourself. Walls are put up in the heart, and then you are not able to receive. Yes, the walls do protect you from situations and people, but the walls also close your heart off. Then you cannot receive the guidance of your intuition; you cannot receive love; and you cannot open to the full joy of life and what is there for you to receive in the moment. You become separated from your Self, shut down to other people, and isolated in your world. These internal wars also create disease within the body as energy gets blocked up.

Self-forgiveness, or forgiveness of anyone else, can only take place when your energy around the situation has become neutralized. With forgiveness, all internal dialogue around the issue is gone, and you can review the situation calmly with no ongoing emotional energy connected to the situation. This is when you begin to gain a true clarity around the truth of the situation. The ego mind dialogue has gone and you can feel the situation with your heart. You are then are able to access learning from the experience—taking responsibility for your part in it. Then you cease to be a victim in the situation, and begin to operate from a powerful place because you have received the teaching—the gift that has come from the issue. This happens when you have personally worked through your true emotional feelings around the situation.

For this to happen you need to give yourself permission to feel whatever is connected to the issue at hand. Be willing to honor whatever feeling is inside of you and allow the full expression of this feeling no matter what it is, remembering that the feeling is not who you are, and the feeling cannot hurt you. You are allowed to feel; you have a right to your feelings, whatever they are.

Open up into your Conscious Breath as you are feeling so that the energy connected to the feeling can leave the cells of your body. Feel them, breathe, and let them go. As you breathe the energy from the emotion can leave the cells of your body, which creates a true resolution inside yourself, and a true freedom from the situation. If we stuff the feelings down, holding the energy inside of us, the energy of the feeling locks into the cells of the body, which creates a congestion in the cells. Then there is no true resolution around the situation because the feelings have not been addressed. Real forgiveness is impossible when this is taking place.

Anger is probably the hardest emotion for us to allow ourselves to feel. There is a social stigma attached to the expression of anger: the unspoken disapproval of expressing anger. People in general are uncomfortable with anger. So you need to be especially aware of allowing yourself to feel all the anger attached to the issue at hand, and give yourself permission to fully feel and express it in the way you need to. It is a powerful moment to just let the build up of anger out and then let go. Your expression of rage or anger does not have to be directed at anyone in particular; you can let it be expressed in an open space by yourself, or with someone neutral who is open to witnessing you while you let it go.

The word *forgiveness* is loaded with guilt, energetically, so you need to begin to open up to a different perspective of the situation, and work toward letting go and healing on very different levels within the issues. There is a strong energy that one *should* forgive—that it is the *right* thing to forgive. Yet in some situations forgiveness may not be possible. If, for instance, we have been badly abused as a child, it may simply be impossible to forgive a parent, but there is a possibility for resolution within yourself for all that happened to you. This is resolution of your own pain, your own anger, or your own sadness from the abuse. Your role is to deal with your own feelings inside. This is what is going to heal you. When we allow this, healing begins to take place within us and we can then move forward in our healing with this parent because we no longer hold such intense feeling connected to the parent. We are not dependant on what our parents may do; we are dependent on ourselves, and our feelings.

The key here is that you must focus on your own feelings, honor those feelings, and know that you do not have to justify what you feel. Once you begin to justify your feelings (this is the ego mind), you negate yourself and what happened to you. There is a true liberation as you give yourself permission to feel. When you feel it all, use the Conscious Breath so it can leave your body, and true healing and resolution can take place.

When we are able to let go of these deep feelings the heart goes through rapid transformation. There is a new sense of freedom and joy. When we hold on to the pain we cannot experience the joy because we are so busy trying to contain the feelings of pain, sadness, and anger. When we get stuck with the belief that we are supposed to forgive we cannot move forward with our healing inside ourselves. We *try* to forgive, but it really gets us nowhere because we don't get to work with our feelings. We are stuck with the ego mind telling us that we are supposed to forgive something or someone.

When you have been hurt in some way your feelings are hurt; this is a truth. How many times have you said to yourself, "Oh, it doesn't matter!"; but it does matter. It matters inside you so much! It is impossible to move into true forgiveness until you have dealt with your own deep feelings within your heart. The pressure to *forgive* can get in the way of you being able to move on and heal in any true way.

With self-forgiveness you develop love, patience, and compassion for yourself. Feel your feelings, and then with love and compassion forgive yourself. You are "perfectly imperfect" as a human being; you are going to make mistakes. Part of our learning here in this lifetime is self-forgiveness. I remind you of the words of Jesus: "When are you going to take yourself off the cross? When are you going to resurrect yourself?" No one else can do it for you.

We spend so much time anchoring ourselves in guilt. When self-reconciliation has taken place, then it is possible for a true forgiveness to take place for the other person or, at the very least, reconciliation within yourself so you are no longer holding on to the energy within the issue. This is what is really important here: to be free from the issue so there can be an energetic release. Guilt is directly connected to the illusion of the third dimension of what you should be and what you should do. When you are immersed in this third-dimensional guilt you are unable to open up and connect to the power of the Self and to move toward what you need to do, and the direction you are supposed to move in your life. Guilt was set up to control—to control mankind to do what they were supposed to do, like being a "good mother," or "doing the right thing," to following society's rules. This is all set up to get you to comply and to be controlled.

The focus on forgiveness is usually on the other person, when in reality the focus first needs to be placed on you and your inner feelings. A much more accurate word for this process is *reconciliation*. Reconciliation requires significant inner work so that you come from the place of a self-healing journey. You can come to terms with, and feel, what has taken place for you. This enables you to let go of the emotional baggage around a person or situation, and be able to deeply heal yourself in the heart. When the heart heals it can be resurrected, and a new level of compassion will be birthed through you.

Then when you begin to live through the compassionate heart, you are able to have that compassion for others. This is another example of the "Divine economy" that moves through your earth plane.

You want to be able to energetically let go of the issues so they no longer trigger emotional reactions within you. Sometimes our work on issues within ourselves is the hardest. We (the ego) judge ourselves so harshly. It is amazing how many things we hold against ourselves. Some of the things that we condemn ourselves for don't even make sense: feelings of guilt, blame, and the words *There must have been something else I could have done; I just know it!* This type of statement is not formed by any reality but comes from the ego mind, based on fear and guilt.

To move yourself out of these cycles, you begin by just being willing to feel, to hold your heart, to hold yourself, and to take a Conscious Breath right into whatever feelings are there. Sometimes, the more you allow yourself to move into the feeling, the more the feeling grows. Just be committed to the feeling and keep the Conscious Breath coming, continuing to be willing to be with whatever feelings are coming up. You don't have to justify the feeling; let it be there. Breath by breath, just feel. Take your time; be patient and loving with yourself.

Sometimes when you are in the middle of this process physical pain begins in some area of your body. This is an emotional issue beginning to move out of your physical body. Your unfelt emotional issues lodge in the cells of your body. Then as you open up to these feelings the emotional congestion begins to leave the cells, and during this process of healing you can sometimes experience that physical pain. Remember that it is leaving your body.

So let's talk about how you work with the pain as it leaves the body. Once you are aware that something is leaving your body, you need to bring your full attention to the site where you are feeling the physical pain. All the body is saying to you with the pain is: Feel here, so this issue can move out of your body now. As you bring your consciousness there, the pain may change: It may get less; it may increase. But as you move toward the pain and feel it, it will begin to leave. Be committed to the pain as completely as you can.

An effective tool is to give the pain a color or a form. As you bring your consciousness to the color or form you take a breath in and out of the mouth. Allow yourself to almost become the texture and the color. Stay with the feeling, and know that nothing will come up in your body that you are not ready to handle. Don't have an agenda; be willing to be with what is presenting.

There are always different levels and layers to the issues that hold in your body, but you do get to the end of it. Some of the issues are set in layers so that we can deal with what we are ready to deal with. When they come up we are able to meet them.

You may feel the need during this process to make a sound. Let the sound move through you and bring it fully into the pain site. Breathe. You may feel as though your body needs to move and to express itself with the movement. Bring your full consciousness into the movement and own this part of your body. It is as though the body is coming back into life and you are receiving back this part of your body. This action is you taking back your power within your body, letting go, and beginning to open up to your responsibility for the self-healing of your physical body.

Bring the focus back to yourself and commit to work through the lessons you have to learn with the issues that are currently in your life. You will begin to have a new level of clarity of what is true, and what is not true, around these issues.

You will be able to open up and take responsibility for the part you have played in each life experience, understanding that you have played a role in each situation. You do not have to take on any one else's part, only to be responsible for yourself. If you find yourself focusing on what the other person's role was, let go, take a breath, and re-focus on yourself. Open up to your feeling in that moment; feel what is happening inside of you.

The key is to ask your self the right questions. The right questions are powerful. Don't be afraid of what the answers may be; just open to the truth in that moment. The truth is always a door to freedom. Once you feel the truth and allow it fully, without judgment, there is something inside you that can just fall away. Hold yourself with love and compassion. You can afford to be compassionate with yourself, and you are allowed to make mistakes; this is a learning process. Let go and breathe.

Some of the questions might be:

Why did I need to draw this experience to myself?

What is my part in this experience?

What do I have to learn in this experience?

What is the pay off for me to stay in this situation?

When you don't emotionally deal with something, you will re-create a similar experience so that you get another opportunity to feel it and heal. This is how the universe works. It keeps bringing you the gift of the lesson so that you have another opportunity to feel it and learn.

I hear people saying, "This just keeps happening again and again," but of course it has to. That's the role of the Universal Consciousness: to give you the opportunity to learn what you have come here to learn. Once you learn the lesson, the cycle stops and you move on. You keep re-creating what you need to learn until you are willing to feel and learn the lesson for your healing. As you heal you become more open and clear about what is taking place in your life and why. You come out of the victim role and begin to play a conscious role in your life.

Self-introspection is an important tool to use to keep aligned with your Self. It's important to do a daily review on what has happened, to assess your experiences and your responses during the day and to reflect on your reactions. It helps you move back into your feelings and have a chance to examine those feelings and reactions in a quiet place. It gives you time to hold yourself with patience, love, and compassion—to gain an understanding of your vulnerabilities and all the different emotional pieces of yourself.

When you hold on to pain, you have to close off your heart. You close off to your heart so you don't feel the pain, but you also close off to feeling anything else and this prevents you from experiencing deep happiness and joy. It's as though you live in a neutral zone, never quite feeling anything deeply, disconnected from yourself and others.

The heart is a receiving tool; it has been designed this way. Through the heart you receive love. Through the heart you receive your abundance on so many levels here on this earth plane.

It takes courage to decide to feel, but as you connect more and more to your heart and open yourself to feel, you will experience the freedom that comes with feeling in the moment. It takes practice to do things differently. It gets easier and easier to get in touch with the real feelings and the real you. As you do, lightness grows within you, and liberation as you take more control and responsibility in each moment.

You have done the very best that you could do up to this moment in time. Forgive yourself for the mistakes you have made and for the decisions you have made along the way that didn't work out the way you expected them to.

This life you have created will begin to make sense as you truly begin to understand the reason for the lessons that life has created for you. Then you can move consciously toward what there is for you to understand or learn in the present moment. It is exciting as you begin to experience yourself in a new powerful way. By embracing yourself, you take ownership of your own creation of your life in each moment. Then you can start co-creating your life in a new way.

Doors will open; Spirit will be with you! And most important, *you* will be with you. This is being alive! Experience the joy and the natural abundance that you have a right to, moving more and more into the flow of the light of the Self. Regain your power, your intuition, and your natural gifts that will take you into living your divine blueprint for this lifetime. Remember who you are in your unlimited self, and open to the abundance and the love that have always been here for you. Experience it fully.

As you open up to more love and compassion for yourself, an amazing thing takes place: Judgments that you have had for others will disappear, and there is a natural feeling of love and compassion. Your heart will expand with that love, love of yourself, and love of others.

And when the love is present, there is no fear.

◇◇◇◇◇◇◇◇◇◇◇◇◇

On the sixth audio track (*www.christinedayonline.com/piol/*) you will be working on self-forgiveness and the transformation of your heart. Open up to the energetic clearing of your heart, allowing the energies of Spirit to assist you. Only you can say *yes* to this process with the Conscious Breath. This is your journey, and I want to remind you that a willingness to receive, transform, and forgive yourself is important.

The breath is also important. It will help with the transformation of the cells in your heart, opening up the cells like flowers to the sun. The breath says two things: "Yes, I am willing to let go," and "Yes, I am willing to receive my light."

I hold the space for you to open up and to be willing to receive the love that is here for you within the energetic realms. We will be transmitting an energetic to assist you in accessing the emotional blocks within the heart so you will be able to access the feeling more completely. As the heart opens and births, you will receive another level of the alignment of the Self and be able to take another step toward reclaiming your place within the Universal whole.

Chapter 7
Journey With the Pleiadians, Within the Stargate Chamber

This next process is in the Stargate chamber, and this journey will create an exciting acceleration of your Self. The Stargate chamber is like a multidimensional womb that has been energetically set up by the Pleiadians so that you can move into another level of initiation with your own light Self. It will take you into a much deeper initiation than up to this point. Within this chamber you will be given access to higher levels of dimensional spaces. Through your experience of this understanding and remembrance you will be able to take your place more completely, with a greater confidence of your place within these spaces. It will open you up to an opportunity to birth yourself to another level of consciousness so that you will begin to remember who you are in your uniqueness. You are ready for this.

Within this initiation you are going to move to a new level of relationship with the Pleiadian energies. It is the time for you to open up to a direct experience with them. This can be done easily within the energies of the Stargate chamber because, as you align with these higher dimensional realms, you expand energetically and can meet the

Pleiadians on a new level. It allows for a clear communication to start between the Pleiadians and you. All communication is done through thought transference. These thought energies transfer effortlessly within the Stargate chamber because there is a pure light form within the chamber. The pure light force activates new areas of your brain for telepathic communication to open up.

This pure light force within the Stargate chamber holds a high frequency of love and the energy initiates into the cells of your body. It's this love element that connects you to your place within the Universal grid. The Pleiadians can meet you within this frequency of love. They vibrate with this loving force, and they will assist you to birth into this pure life force and into this frequency of love. Your cells will be bathed with this pure life force of love, creating a birth within each cell. The Pleiadians will assist you in an integration process so that your cells can move into a rapid adjustment from this new energy. This integration allows an even more complete ability for you to be able to communicate with them, as you align with the quality of this loving force from the Stargate chamber. You will be able to form a deeper, more personal relationship with them because your personal expansion into the light brings you deeper into the oneness, and the Pleiadians are a part of this oneness.

Part of the Pleiadians' role is to hold these energetic dimensional platforms open for you, and as they hold them open you will be able to move and flow into these initiation spaces. The cells of your body will be energetically aligned with higher levels of your light. The Pleiadians will witness you as you move through your different initiating levels, as you birth yourself. They will continue to hold the platform open so that you can become aligned with the expanded dimensional spaces of the Stargate chamber. They will not interfere with you in these initiations; their commitment is to witness you and continue to hold the energetic platforms for you, helping you anchor the fourth-, fifth-, and sixth-dimensional energies on our planet.

This is an important process—the transformation of moving from a third-dimensional planet to the fourth-, fifth-, and sixth-dimensional planet. The work you are going to be doing here in the Stargate journeys will assist in the transformation of your energies. This transformation of yourself is incredibly powerful for the whole planet as you take more of your place within the Universe whole. Your new energies will be able to automatically transmit a higher frequency out through the planet, assisting with the new levels of energy that need to be anchored on the earth plane at this time.

The Stargate is an energetic multidimensional space, but there is a stable place within the Stargate, where you can journey on many different levels and move into multidimensional levels of initiation. It has been created by the Pleiadians for you to initiate into your light at an accelerated rate. The Pleiadians work directly with you within the Stargate; you cannot do this alone because you need the Pleiadians to open up the entry point for you. Three Pleiadians will hold you energetically so that you can enter the Stargate chamber, and they will assist you in your initial opening up to the vast energies that can be accessed within the chamber. Because of the stability that has been created in the Stargate, you have the means to take yourself there with the help of the Pleiadians. They will help you learn to work within the multidimensional energetic spaces, and connect with the different aspects of your multidimensional self. An important part of these journeys is to reconnect to these aspects of your multidimensional self and to access energetic tools so that you can utilize them now in this lifetime. The Pleiadians will help you in these re-connections, as you are ready.

You will learn to navigate yourself through these multidimensional spaces, and with each journey to open to the Truth and love there. With each experience you will anchor yourself more to this reality and be able to access this loving truth in your daily life here on this earth plane.

You are always held by the Pleiadians in the Stargate processes, and they will be monitoring you energetically, making sure that you are able to integrate the energies you are opening up and into. They will make sure that you do not overextend yourself within these energetic levels. As you move into and expand deeper within the Stargate's many dimensional openings you will find a new level of alignment to yourself, and a new sense of ease and peace flowing through your consciousness. You will bring these energies back with you from these dimensional journeys and as you integrate them through your energetic field and cells of your body they will automatically transfer and impact your day-to-day living.

There are aspects of your Self that flourish within these dimensional energies, and the energies that you encounter on these journeys will open up within you an ability to self-heal on a physical, emotional, and spiritual level.

It's important that you drink plenty of water to hydrate your cells before the journey. Your cells increase in vibration as you open up into these expanded light experiences, activating a quickening within the cell structure, which creates a friction within the cell, so that heat begins to build with this higher vibration of light. Drinking water helps the cells more easily integrate the new level of light that you will be opening up to when you begin to initiate within these dimensional spaces. Being hydrated also helps you take in more of your expanded energies of light more easily and flow energetically with these dimensional spaces.

Also drink a lot of water after your experience in the Stargate, when you have completed your journey, to help your body fully integrate and adjust to the transformational energy that has been activated through your system. Remember that this energy that you have initiated into is your own light: the expanded light energy of the Self that has come into your cells. This light will directly affect your ability to feel more anchored and centered in your Self; it will bring you into a more deeper awareness of your connection to the life force that exists within your world and your place within it. Your awareness of the Pleiadians and the Spiritual energies will increase in your day-to-day life here on the planet, and you will be able to utilize their help as you take new steps forward in your life.

There are many other light beings and masters that you may personally work with. The Stargate energy is an aspect of the Oneness, and the Pleiadians work in conjunction with all light forms within this space. The Oneness is all that exists, and all the energetic light forms work together within the high level of light and exquisite quality of love that exist within the Stargate dimensional spaces. You are going to be initiated into being a more conscious part of this Oneness—to take your place being more consciously aligned to the spiritual realms as you journey here.

You are going to be given a team of Pleiadian energies that will work with you in your initiating processes as you take your journey with the seventh online audio track. Their commitment is to work with you within the Stargate chamber and at any other time that you ask for their help.

The Pleiadians' hope is that you will build a relationship with them—an alliance so they can continue to assist you to unfold on many different initiation levels outside of the Stargate chamber. During each journey they will hold energetic spaces for you to unfold into, and assist you in your ongoing initiations, helping you integrate the energies from each specific journey. They are willing to stay with you as a team and are committed to assist you as you do your work in the world, if that is what you want.

Before you begin your journey you are being asked to open up into a state of receivership. You need to do this consciously, by taking responsibility and saying, "Yes, I open to receive this initiation." Claim your Self, your birthright to receive and your power. Open up into your heart, so that you breathe into your heart and your cells open in a full state to receive your Self.

You are being asked to let go of everything that is here in the third-dimensional space during this initiation journey, and be willing to allow yourself to unfold. Allow yourself to open to what is here for you within this journey. It's the time to do this: to reclaim your place and to allow the space of the Stargate to bring you into a new state of your Self. It's time to birth into a new aspect of *you*—to open to a new dimensional aspect of yourself, reclaiming you.

This journey begins in the same Formation as described in Chapter 3. However, you will not be working with any other people in this Formation. A team of Pleiadian energies will take three Formation places. The fourth place in the Formation will be your place. They will hold you energetically as you take this journey into the Stargate dimensions, and create specific energetic spaces that allow you to enter the Stargate realms.

You are going to begin by activating the Base in the same way as you did in Chapter 3. Once the Base is activated you will be taken by the three Pleiadian energies into an energetic Stargate chamber.

The Stargate exists in a very different dimensional space than the Formation. It holds a much higher level of energetic light and is linked to the Universal grid. Within the Stargate is the Stargate chamber, a placed filled with light. This is where your initiations will take place. It is a stable energetic place where you will be able to easily integrate the birthing energy of a new dimensional aspect of yourself.

After the initiations are complete the Pleiadian energies will bring you back to the Formation base, where you will integrate the new aspects of yourself into the cells of the heart. I will also be with you energetically as you take this journey. Spirit will be with you. We will all be witnessing you, and celebrating you in this birth!

◇◇◇◇◇◇◇◇◇◇◇◇

I want to open you up to the new energies of this initiation that are going to be on this seventh track (*www.christinedayonline.com/piol/*). Have a great journey!

Chapter 8
Manifesting Through the Sacred Heart

It is time for you to begin to open up to your own manifesting abilities. Manifesting is a natural a part of your divine abilities to develop in this lifetime, on this earth plane. You have forgotten who you are and what you are capable doing. The ability to *manifest* is something you have forgotten about, something you need to *remember*. The ability to manifest is your natural gift that you have and have always had. This process of remembering is not learning anything new, but an awakening of yourself and taking back your power, moving toward yourself and opening up into this ability to manifest.

Manifesting involves taking back the responsibility to co-create your life and taking responsibility in receiving your creation. It is an understanding that you deserve to have abundance in your life as a part of your natural birthright so that you can now open up to receive the life you want to create for yourself.

Not having enough is one of the biggest illusions of the third-dimensional plane. Your belief in "lack" keeps you in a powerless place. You have being playing this victim role for lifetimes. Now it is time to wake up and to claim your right to manifest now.

When I talk about abundance on all levels I refer to:

> **Financial abundance:** You have a right to all the financial abundance that you wish. Know that your abundance has nothing to do with anyone else's natural abundance; you cannot take too much. Your abundance is unlimited; each one of you decides when you are ready to receive this abundance for yourselves.

> **Physical health:** Your physical health plays an important part in the quality of life that you can lead. Part of the manifesting process is manifesting healthy cells, so that you can be physically strong, and your cells can and will vibrate with a new alignment to the light of the Self, and be a part of the universal pulse or heartbeat. As this new alignment begins to take place, there will be a new sense of well-being within your body.

> **Emotional abundance of love:** Create an abundance of love in your life, to be able to receive the love and support of the universe as well as opening up to loving relationships with other people—relationships with people that are balanced with respect, and anchored with deep connections through the heart. Part of the manifesting process is to bring you into an alignment with these energetics so that you can begin to draw these deep connections of the heart toward yourself.

All manifestation is done through a connection to your sacred heart. You have worked with many processes to clear the heart, align with the heart, and begin to consciously live through the heart. Now you are ready to become a conscious co-creator of your world It's a huge step, and it brings such freedom to you.

Through your sacred heart you are going to connect with your passion and your heart's desire. It's important that as you open up to what it is that you want to create in your life, that you also open up to receive the living energetic of your creation. You must receive this "living energetic of your creation" through your sacred heart. By "your living energetic of your creation" I mean that whatever you want to create, whatever you wish for yourself, has an energetic pattern to it. It's a living energetic. So once you know what your creation will be, you will notice its energetic pattern. You may sense this energy, see this energy, or feel this energy. It does not matter how it presents itself to you. All things that are created begin with this living energetic. Once it is established it can be anchored on this earth plane. *Your* manifestation process activates this living energetic. As you design what you want for yourself, an energetic blueprint is formed within the Universe. And as you bring your consciousness to that blueprint and bring it into your sacred heart, it becomes activated—a living energetic. Then it becomes possible for it to anchor in a physical form in your life.

It takes courage to open to this energy, because its activation connects to the passion of your heart. It is alive, and you are going to have to meet this passionate energy through your heart as it is created. It's as though the heart begins to get excited as you begin to live with this new energy of the activation of your passion. The heart actually expands with the energy of your creation, and there is a new part of your life force that moves through the cells of the heart. This energy is the light of the Self. The heart is going to go through rapid transformation, and there is a quickening throughout the body as the manifesting begins to be activated.

These are the steps you need to take to enter this process:

1. The most important first step is to look carefully, in close detail, at the life you are now living. This is the life you have created for yourself up to this point.

2. You need to own your creation. This means you need to take responsibility for your creation. Until you are willing to take responsibility for past creations, you will not be able to begin manifesting a new blueprint for your future. It is essential that you own what you have created and to own every piece.

3. Begin actively participating in your life, reviewing what you have created for yourself moment by moment. The clarity of why you have created certain situations comes from the connection of the Self through the heart, knowing that you needed each experience, and that each experience has brought you to this very moment. You need to be open to all the parts you played in your creation and the lessons your creation has brought to you.

4. Then you need to give thanks to yourself for the teaching you have received, and the lessons you have learned. Give thanks for what you have created and acknowledge yourself for needing these experiences.

5. You need to spend time being with this creation of yours, holding yourself with compassion, love, and patience as you take the time to fully examine what you have been living and what you created for yourself up to this point. This is a very powerful step, and it's important not to rush the process. Some of it may be painful, but don't push away from the pain; just breathe and allow yourself to visit each moment. Each piece, in each moment, needs to be held in a very sacred way. Feel yourself, feel the journey, and breathe.

Once you have reviewed your life, hold your sacred heart with your hand and allow yourself to open to your heart's desire for your life now. Feel the areas of your life that need to change—the areas you have created for yourself that no longer serve you. *You* can make the changes now. Be aware you do not have to do this on your own. You are in the flow of the light of the Self through the sacred heart. You can let go, and allow that aspect of Self to assist you in opening up those opportunities and new experiences to you that you are ready for now.

At this time in the process you need to pay particular attention to the part of you that may not feel it deserves more. This part of the ego mind needs to understand that you have done the best you could in the life you have lived up to this point. Mistakes have been made, and mistakes are a natural part of any learning process.

Mistakes are inevitable in our lives, made through the act of just being human. They are not acts designed to harm another; they are just acts that create something, a ripple going out into the world. These ripples are designed to move outward, opening up experiences for other people so that they can have their human experience.

Let go of the guilt and the shame, the self-accusations of not being perfect, and the mistakes that have been made. Turn toward yourself in love, holding yourself with compassion. Open up to be willing to turn toward yourself in an act of forgiveness. Let go of that illusion of perfection, and begin loving that aspect of your human self. Turn back toward yourself in an act of loving embrace and come back into those words *I am.*

It's important to be conscious of the illusions in the reality of third-dimensional illusion as you live them, stepping back and watching as these illusions play out in your world, like you are watching a play on a stage, playing your part. Be grateful for being here at this time and being consciously aware of the illusions here on this planet.

As you commit to feeling and healing yourself from your internal wounds that you have received by being human here on this earth plane, open to the depth of your feeling and honor that feeling. The feeling can then leave the body and we can set ourselves free on another level. Be willing to understand the truth about your journeys, and the truth about your life: that you came to have experiences but not to hold on to the issues. You came just for the experience itself as it happened. You were never meant to hold on to the pain, blame, and guilt; just have the experience, feel it, and let go.

Take a breath, to say yes to letting go of your story, and to all the pieces of yourself that played throughout the stories and that made up your life.

You have a right to move on, and allow more for yourself now. You are allowed to receive. It is your divine right to receive.

It's Time to Move On!

It's time to activate a blueprint for yourself to manifest what it is that you want for yourself in this life. What is your heart's desire?

Open consciously to your heart and breathe. Leave the ego mind while you connect into your sacred heart. Bring your hand down to hold the physical heart, and then bring your full consciousness to your hand, feel the pressure of your hand, and breathe. Close your eyes, and just allow all of your energy and consciousness to come into the heart.

Keep your eyes closed and just breathe, allowing the energy to build through the sacred heart, and the energy of the blueprint to activate through the heart and expand through the cells. As you allow the most detailed description of what you want to manifest to expand and flow through the heart, you will feel new levels of energy build around this manifestation. The manifestation begins to birth itself, through the heart and then into your world.

There are no limits to how big your manifestation can be; allow the full picture to form. It may feel as though this manifestation has a life of its own as the heart begins to expand and connect to this project. The energy of the Self connects directly to the heart. This energy building is the activation of your manifestation of the Self.

It is not important to know how this manifestation is going to take place. The light of your Self is the director, and the Universal Consciousness will assist in the manifestation of your energetic blueprint. You don't need to know the details or how you are going to manifest what it is that you want. Once you open to your heart's desire and begin to build the energetic blueprint, you can let go and witness the manifestation to take place.

As this blueprint begins to be birthed on this earth plane, your life force will expand through your cells because you will be living passionately. You have always been meant to live in this passionate way. With this passion in your life you are truly alive. Claim your abundance. You cannot take too much; it is unlimited in form.

You are not meant to struggle in your life. I know this is hard to believe; what you see around you is struggle. Struggle is a strong third-dimensional belief that has played out on this planet for lifetimes. Struggle and fear, struggle and fear—this is a pattern of strong ego belief that has been very active on the earth plane, and it's your ego that has kept you in this pattern by its limitation.

The time for the ego to rule is over for you. You will find ease in your life, as you let go and allow yourself to move with the flow of abundance that will open up in your life as the activation of your blueprint is made manifest in your world.

"How can this be so simple?" you ask. By letting go and simply allowing the Self to take you in each moment. You are being asked to open and allow the miracles to take place in your life. Open to the wonderment of each moment, and allow yourself to receive the abundance. You deserve this abundance; you are worthy to receive all that is rightfully yours with ease and grace. Just let go, knowing you are perfect the way you are in this moment.

Open your heart up now, hold your heart, and take a breath. Be aware of us holding you with so much love. You have so much courage; you have come so far. We hold you in this moment in great love and regard.

Each one of us has a responsibility on this earth plane to open up and live our divine aspect. Each one of us is unique, and that uniqueness is needed here, *now!* It's about being all that you are, and having a willingness and courage to live it, allowing it to take you where you need to go. Have the courage to step forward and open up to what you need to be doing in your life, living your passion, and being in the flow.

When you are in the flow, doors open effortlessly.

As you activate your heart's desire of manifesting, the heart can expand more and more. The heart is connected to the soul. It has the ability to lead you to your soul's desire. The more you are prepared to live through your heart and activate the manifesting potential of yourself, the more you are going to experience your passion and your true mission. Open up to where you belong in the world. Draw to you the people that you need to support you on your unique journey—what I call your "soul family."

To Begin to Form What You Want for Your Life

1. Move your breath into your physical body, away from your head, into the vicinity of your physical heart. Formulate what you want for your life, what you want to manifest in your life, and how you want that life to look. Be specific.

2. Do not concern yourself with the details of how this is going to unfold. Do not try to think about what to do next; it will not give you the right answers. The mind does not have the answers to take you on this journey. It will keep you in a cycle of sameness and frustration. Connecting through the sacred heart will give you the answers you need. If the ego mind is creating doubt just bring your consciousness into the heart and breathe. You will begin to feel the truth and calmness again.

3. Stay physically connected to the heart during this process; hold your heart and take a Conscious Breath as you map out what it is you are going to manifest.

4. Don't limit yourself to what you can have. Allow yourself to open to your abundance fully.

This will restructure your life in a positive way, bringing change where there needs to be change, and expanding relationships and things in your life that resonate with the truth of where you need to go. It will support your needs—the needs of your heart: the true needs of the Self. It's you feeding you, with the spiritual food of the Self.

The only things that will disappear will be people and things that don't truly serve you and that are not based on any real authenticity for you. When you begin to live the true life for yourself, you automatically are present in the moment. Being in the moment brings you out of a separated state. You will no longer be alone. You will become much more present for yourself, and then automatically more present for people around you.

As you begin to live toward a wholeness and truth, there is a new authenticity—not perfection, but commitment to the truth. You align with a new integrity in your life and experience great changes. The activation of your energetic blueprint that you are going to manifest will bring you into these alignments. It is time for you to open up to this full state of receivership. All of this is yours; it has always been here waiting for you.

Your world will come to meet you as you align with the rhythm of the universe. Your heartbeat will begin aligning with the universal heartbeat. You will recognize Truth—not your truth but universal Truth.

This does not mean there will not be challenges along the way, but you will flow with these challenges and you will not be meeting them alone. You will experience a newly found strength and understanding for whatever your particular mission is on this earth plane. Living like this creates an enormous re-balancing on the earth plane, and you will be playing your part.

When you work with the heart's desire you automatically go with the flow. It is so important not to force anything into action. When it is the right direction and the right time you will experience things falling into place effortlessly. Where there is resistance, do not push or try to force a result. Simply let go, knowing that it is either not the time or simply not where you need to go. When an opportunity opens up, when the door opens, walk through. If you use this rule you will stay in the flow, and you will be taken where you need to go to move to your next step. You can trust it.

Don't be attached to how you are going to get to where you want to go, how it is going to look, or work out. Just trust! Let go of the mind and allow the heart to take you. The energy of the Self will divinely orchestrate your new life, as it does its job, manifesting your blueprint in your life.

The inspiration of Spirit is beyond what the human mind can know, recognize, or understand, so *trust* is a very important factor. It is imperative to develop trust within our humanness. The more you are willing to trust, the more Spirit can step forward and assist you in the miracle of your life. You cannot listen to Spirit one day, and not the next. You need to follow through on all directives given, so that you can be taken where you need to go to achieve your manifesting goal. There is no point in asking help from Spirit and then, when this guidance is given, choosing the steps that suit you but not following the others. This way will not get you to where you want to go. You need to follow completely or not at all. You must trust, or not—this is your choice— moment by moment, step by step. Only you can find the answers for yourself. You do have help from the spiritual realms—tremendous help—and a constant love surrounding you.

It is up to you to continue to open up to this love through your heart, allow it to transform you, and heal you from lifetimes of pain. Allow an unlimited abundance of support and love into your life, and into the cells of your body. It is time for this, and it is your natural birthright for you to have it. You do not have to earn the right to this love; you don't have to change anything about yourself to have it right now. You are enough just as you are!

You Are Enough!

Breathe and take this Truth in. The love that is present for you at any one time is unlimited. All you have to do is reach out and open up to access this profound love. Remember that you can only access it through your heart.

The human being has a problem accepting the simplicity of this truth. Lifetimes of conditioning and self-judgment have kept you separate from this love. You basically don't believe you deserve to be loved in this way. Only by linking into the heart are you going to be able to receive just how precious you are; to be able to return to your innocence and to be able to re-experience this innocence and feel safe enough to open to your vulnerability and live it.

Vulnerability does not mean that you are weak. It brings you into a place of strength and clarity that allows you to stand close to Spirit, and close to your own sacred heart—to the truth and remembrance of who you really are. It links you back to the unlimited gifts of your divine Self, and allows you to begin to use these gifts now in this lifetime.

◇◇◇◇◇◇◇◇◇◇◇◇

It is now the time to listen to the eighth audio track (*www. christinedayonline.com/piol/*), which is designed to activate the manifesting process through the sacred heart. Prepare yourself with something you want to begin to manifest in your life, before you listen to the track.

Know that we will be with you on this journey to assist you, and to witness your initiation into the Sacred heart as you activate your manifesting blueprint. We will witness you in the activation of your heart's desire, and support this energy and you as it anchors onto the earth plane.

Be aware as you work with this manifesting blueprint, it is possible to make changes and adjustments to what you are manifesting at any time. Be as creative in your designs as you need to be, and allow the creation energy to flow through you. This is a fluid project, and it's important that you learn to flow with it. You flow and become a true part of it. It's as though there is no separation between what you are manifesting, your heart, and you. Honor this creative energy and honor yourself. Bring your uniqueness to the design of what you want for yourself. Be flamboyant in your design! Allow you heart to express itself; don't hold back with this passion. Give to yourself. Then activate your passionate energy through the heart!

Please open track 8. Remember to let go and allow your full creation to move through your heart. We are with you. We celebrate your emancipation from the third-dimensional limitations.

Chapter 9

Expanding Your Initiation Into the Sacred Pyramid's Energy Within the Formation

I want to acknowledge you for moving into this chapter. Before you is another aspect of the Formation initiations. These initiations will bring you into deeper dimensional levels within the Sacred Pyramid energies. These energies are powerful and transformational.

It is really important that you focus on being in the moment as you journey into these deeper dimensional levels of the Sacred Pyramid. Remember that when you open fully into the moment you automatically move out of separation. So as you stay in the moment this means that you are fully aligned to *now*, not thinking of the past or the present, but bringing your consciousness into the gift that is before you in this moment, allowing yourself to fully receive the energies and experiences that are before you. You will then be able to meet these new expanded spaces in a personal and intimate way. There is a unique pathway held open for each one of you within these sacred journeys so you can access your personal space by staying present with each breath, and activate the pathways with your consciousness as they open up to you. Because you have to consciously say *yes* to each unique opening, you must be present to do so. You are taking your place one more time: one more conscious step toward your self. The Pleiadians are responsible for creating these openings, and you are ready for these personalized openings. It is through your connection to your Sacred heart that you will connect into these specific initiations and experience.

You are being asked to stay in a fluid state as you begin your journey. This will allow you to open up to the flow within the spaces that will open within the Sacred Pyramid. You are going to be asked to step forward and take your place within the Sacred Pyramid. As you consciously do this, it will allow your energetic place to emerge within this space. You are going to find your unique place within this opening. Now it is up to you to allow yourself to become one with this space.

Let's talk about how you move into this state of oneness. The desire is important, as is your being conscious within the space and taking a breath, but as you do this let go of all that exists within your third-dimensional world. You need to let go for a few moments to allow a full union to take place between you and this energetic space. This makes it possible for you to reclaim these energies and integrate them into your cells.

What you are allowing by doing this is an acceptance of a multi-dimensional aspect of yourself, reclaiming yourself on another level and anchoring this expanded aspect of you into the cells of your body. This is going to allow you to utilize these energies within your life here on the earth plane now. You will be able to move into a deeper flow with your Self through your heart and to birth yourself into a deeper inspiration of your sacred heart. So don't forget to bring your hands to your chest and breathe so that you can be right in your body and connected fully into the heart while your heart goes through another level of transformation.

There are many journeys to take here; each one opens up to you a different unique journey through your place within the Sacred Pyramid. As you work with the audio tracks more than once, each journey will be different. Don't look for the same experiences. Each journey is uniquely set up for you, and each journey is important for its different content and multidimensionality. The ego mind might try to re-create an experience from your last journey; you don't want this to happen. Bring your consciousness to your heart and be in the heart for your journey.

As you connect to the Sacred Pyramid you will begin to understand a new level of awareness of your ability to create within the universe and to navigate yourself on a whole new level with the life force energy that is within you. The work in the Sacred Pyramid will help you utilize your own life force energies, manifesting and working with your passionate self as a co-creator. You reclaim aspects of yourself and realign yourself with your personal power. As you expand and develop your skills of being in the moment, your own awareness takes you into new experiences.

Because *time* is one of the greatest illusions of this third dimension, each frame of each moment is unlimited in its ability to take you into deeper and deeper experiences. These dimensional spaces are timeless. As you bring your consciousness into an experience and take a breath, you will find that your experiences begin to expand, change, or deepen. Just let go into the expansion, and allow yourself to flow into the energy or experience that is present. You do this by bringing your attention to the energy or experience, letting go, and breathing, bringing your focus deeper into what is happening. It does not matter how subtle your experience is. You can open as easily into a subtle experience as you can into an intense experience.

It may feel as though you have been gone for hours or days as you enter a dimensional space within the Sacred Pyramid. And yet you come back from this journey a short time later, according to our earth time. Because there is no *time,* you are able to have an experience within the Sacred Pyramid, and then at a later date bring your consciousness back to that moment and continue to work with that same experience, expanding it out on many other levels. Once you have entered a dimensional space, and have initiated and anchored the energies into your cells, it allows you to re-enter this space at any time. This is an important point to understand: You can revisit any experience and allow yourself to fully integrate all aspects of your experience at a deeper level. It does not matter how long ago you had the experience, because time does not truly exist. You can always re-utilize these connections. There is great value in revisiting powerful experiences because there are always new levels of the experiences that you can receive and initiate into. As you are ready for new levels, you can receive deeper initiations. You are not alone when you re-enter these dimensional spaces; the Pleiadians and Spiritual forces will always be with you, supporting you in expanded initiations.

The Sacred Pyramid energy has a series of powerful sacred geometrical dimensional spaces. Actually they are entry points for you to initiate into. To enter these openings simply bring your consciousness into the experience you are having and let go, allowing yourself to flow into what is happening. You will breathe and bring your full focus into the experience. This will move you to the entry of the doorway and will connect you to your initiation experience. You have a place within this Sacred Pyramid, and it is for you to find and take your place within this space.

As you move into this space and consciously take your place you will open up to an almost familiar space. It may feel powerful and expanded as you assume your place. You rejoin an aspect of your energy and there may be sacred tools available here for you to reconnect to. The energy of these tools can be accessed now so that you can utilize the power of them in your life. As you move into these powerful aspects of yourself you will receive a download of this energy into the cells. You will begin to open to new alignments of yourself through the different levels of initiation that are available within these dimensional spaces set in the Pyramid. It's important that you anchor the energy that you bring back from each journey into the cells of your body. To do this you simply bring your hands to your chest and take a Conscious Breath through the cells. You need to continue to do this until you can feel the breath moving through your body. This energy that you bring back from the journey in the pyramid is an aspect of your own light Self. Each of these journeys will create an acceleration of your awakening.

You will be realigned back into your Self. Each journey will bring you into another level of the Self, and it will bring the physical body to another level of transformation and healing.

Each time you take another journey with the audio tracks you will have a very different experience (because you are different), and each time you complete the journey you bring another level of your light back into the cells. These journeys are continual birthing opportunities that are made available for you. It is exciting and wonderful!

When you are in the Sacred Pyramid energy it is important to open to each moment and be open to the energy that is present for you. It is essential to keep the breath flowing, slowly and consciously. Just place your hand on your chest and feel that breath; *be that breath.* Let go. Each time you open fully to the moment you open and anchor more of yourself.

Remember: The breath says *yes* to the moment— "Yes, I am willing to open into a full state of receivership." You give your permission with that *yes* breath—permission for the Pleiadian energies to assist you in downloading your initiating energies into your cells, moment by moment, breath by breath. The Pleiadians are energetically monitoring you, so that you cannot take in too much energy for your systems. This will allow you to open and fully expand into these initiating energies, knowing you are being fully assisted and monitored so you can open to the full initiation.

Consciously opening in this way to each moment brings you into a state of Oneness with all things, and moves you out of separation. Each individual experience of each moment moves you to a new level and awakening of alignment to yourself, and to your flow within the Universal Consciousness. It actually aligns you more completely to that flow of Oneness.

If you begin to work with this process a few moments a day in the beginning, you will find yourself moving into this deeper state of awareness naturally. This is returning you back to your natural state of oneness, and it's in this state of each moment that you can re-align with all your natural gifts.

This process of initiation, of opening to your power within the Pyramid is going to allow you to be more present in your day-to-day life. It will bring you more completely into your experiences, because you will find yourself aligning more naturally into each moment. Your life will take on a more brilliant form. Your awareness of your connection to yourself will expand; everything will appear richer, and fuller in some way. There is so much more for you to experience here on a daily basis in each experience. When you are truly open to the moment, living your experiences, you will find a new level of life force with all things, and you will be aligned with that life force.

Being willing to open to the moment is going to be very important with this next group of audio files. In these tracks you will be opening to the Formation base, as in Chapter 3.

There is going to be a sacred patterning for you to open up to within the Pyramid. Be aware that this sacred patterning is uniquely yours. It is a type of energetic blueprint that will activate through all your cells, awakening you to another level of yourself. It will open up new energies within the body so that you will more easily recognize your mission here in this lifetime.

Let go and allow yourself to experience yourself on another level as completely as you can as you work within the Pyramid's dimensional energies. Open to the support and love of the Universe as you open up to your initiation's here.

◇◇◇◇◇◇◇◇◇◇◇◇

Now open the ninth audio track (*www.christinedayonline.com/piol*). Have a great journey.

Chapter 10
Belonging to the Whole, to the Oneness

You are now ready to begin another level of your journey. This journey will give you access to your place within the Collective Consciousness. I liken the Collective Consciousness to a huge ocean, made up of billions and billions of drops of water. Each drop of water is a unique divine aspect of the whole, and you are a drop of that water. Within that drop you have a unique divine aspect that makes you part of that whole ocean—within this Collective Consciousness.

It is the time for you to take another step forward and move into another alignment with your Self. It is about claiming your place—claiming your uniqueness with a conscious action. This is taking your power back, making the statement *I am*. This is part of the Self Healing Prophecy: that you are to take back your power by consciously taking your place at this time, realigning yourself to your divine aspect within your place on the Universal grid, which is in essence the Collective Consciousness. As you begin to take a more conscious role of the existence of your place you are able to anchor this alignment energetically through your cells. You are then able to live with these new alignments, bringing you into a more conscious aspect of your Self as you live here on this earth plane.

As you move back to an alignment of your place within the Universal grid, you begin to remember aspects of your role here, and what you have come here to achieve. This grid is really like a huge light wheel where each of us within the universe has our place, and part of our journey is to reconnect back to our place on the Universal grid. As you realign, your place on the light wheel your place on the grid begins to activate and pulsate with light. This light then begins to activate your unique signature outward into the Universe.

As you align back to your place on the grid, you then can begin transmitting out a brilliance that is uniquely yours. You are able to consciously work and channel this energy of the Self through your physical body on this earth plane. This will help you to live with an understanding of what you have come to do in this lifetime, and give you the tools that you need to complete this journey. It will also give you access to consciously connect and utilize the help from the spiritual and energetic realms, so that you will be able to work as part of an energetic team.

Your connection to your place on the grid is a step-by-step process of your awakening to your Self. Know that there are ongoing alignments that will continue to take place on the Universal grid, as you are ready to energetically receive more aspects of your Self.

Your place waits for you to connect on a *conscious* level. This means that you need to start to be aware of your alignment and place within the Universal grid. Then you can begin to move your energy— your conscious awareness—outward. As you begin to open up to your unique place on the grid you will remember aspects of yourself. You will then be able to experience a deeper understanding and sense of yourself on a human level as well as becoming re-tuned to the spiritual nature of yourself.

A natural self-compassion and love for yourself will open up as you start to be aware of these two aspects of yourself, and most importantly you will feel your humanness and understand yourself in the aspect of being human on this earth plane at this time, and appreciate the courage it has taken you to be here, because you will no longer be condemning yourself for your life, but be able to appreciate the journey you have taken up to this point. This conscious movement toward activating your place on the grid is a large part of your awakening. When you align consciously toward your place on the grid you will connect to a new level of your intuition, because you are lining up with this higher aspect of the Self, which is part of the Collective Consciousness. All knowledge is accessed through this space and accessible to you in this space.

The ego mind has tremendous resistance to the Collective Consciousness, but if you move down into your heart you can feel the truth of it. Stay in your heart during this process; hold your hand on your divine heart and breath. Allow this for yourself now!

You have stayed small for so long, believing yourself to be something so limited, and because of this all of your natural abilities have shut down. It has linked you into the third-dimensional *illusion of lack, struggle, and powerlessness.* The ego mind holds us strongly within the third-dimensional illusion, so it's essential to allow yourself to change this habit of holding onto the mind.

When I talk of natural abilities, remember that I speak of our ability to create; our ability to self-heal; our natural birthright to have unlimited abundance on all levels; and our unlimited energy that we can draw from within ourselves; and to be able to connect into the multidimensional aspect of the Self.

The Universe celebrates as you take your place because your energy is necessary for true union—for the jigsaw to be complete. Activating your place within the grid makes a difference!

As you consciously take your place on the Universal grid, the cells in your body begin to go through a transformation with the connection to this new light aspect. Each cell in your body has a transmitter, and the quickening process activates this transmitter in each cell so you begin to draw toward you different energetic experiences in this world and in your life. Because your new vibration attracts higher levels of energetic experience, they come in the form of new levels of abundance moving into your world.

This transmitter within the cell has been dormant until now. The transmitter begins to vibrate as you open up on a conscious level to your place within the grid and begins to assist you in anchoring you more completely into that place. This is an exciting and monumental step for you. It is about you accessing another level of your power. It brings you into an alignment with the Truth and Knowledge within the Universe, and allows you to anchor it in your life on new levels. It's like you are now hooked up to a strong cable connection, and finally you will be able to receive a new clarity and understanding of your life. This allows you to move very differently in the world.

The understanding and clarity from your connection to the Universal grid allow you to move and be in the world, while at the same time be connected to the Spiritual realms and the Collective Consciousness. You will be held in a loving embrace as you live, able to move with the oneness of all living things on this planet. The support of this will hold you as you anchor the love here on the earth, and this alignment will greatly assist you on your journey here this lifetime.

Without this *conscious* activation, your cells cannot activate the transmitter to the Self. You have free will on this earth plane: You must choose the moment that you wish to begin this level of awakening. We cannot interfere; we do not wish to interfere. This awakening has been made possible at this time because of the Self Healing Prophecy that was activated January 2009. We hold the space for you to unfold and awaken now.

All that is required is for you to open to the possibility of the truth that your place does exist within the Universal Consciousness—that you have a place. It must be activated through your heart. As you open up to that possibility, you bring your consciousness upward toward your place and take a breath, claiming your place. As you do this there will be an activation of the transmitters within your cells, and they will begin this alignment with the Universal Consciousness. You can do this. You have nothing to lose and everything to gain. Empower yourself; take the Self back. Claim yourself.

You have already connected to your unique place on some level, but now it is time to begin to move into a more complete alignment to this place of Self. It's going to be a step-by-step process, taking you to a deeper and deeper place within you. As you move forward and take this next step, the energy within your cells will begin to pulse and expand. This is light—*your light.* The connection of this light within the cells brings an awakening to you: an awakening of universal truth, and a new clarity within you of that truth.

You will begin to receive guidance that is clear and accurate. You will receive an understanding of yourself, and the journey of your life up to this point, and the importance of all that you have experienced in your journey.

As you link to the unlimited knowledge that exists within the Universal Consciousness, you begin an accelerated awakening that connects you to a new level of creativity within you—divine creativity that is connected to the love element in all life force. You will be uniquely you, flowing as part of the love that exists within the Ocean of Light within the Collective Consciousness.

As you enter into this ocean of consciousness you will become even more defined within your unique signature of your divine nature. There will be no sense of you losing your Self within this Ocean of Light. To the contrary, you will experience a more complete aspect of yourself. There will be a new clarity, which will give you a much more defined experience of who you are and a deeper sense of your place on this planet.

From the earth plane you will flourish as you take your place within the Universal Consciousness, holding so many unique energies and abilities from which you will unfold into. You will become a beacon of the light in the world, transmitting out your unique signature of light!

◇◇◇◇◇◇◇◇◇◇◇◇

Pleiadian Initiations of Light

The 10th audio track (*www.christinedayonline.com/piol/*) is designed to take you on an unlimited journey to anchor you within your place in the Universal Consciousness, within the Ocean of Light. Every time you listen to these tracks the transmitters in your cells of your body will become increasingly aligned with your unique place within the Universal Consciousness. Take your place. Choose the moment now to activate your awakening on this level. I will be with you energetically; the Pleiadians will be with you if you call them forward to be there. My love is with you as you take this journey!

Chapter 11
Physical Healing Through the Cells

It is now time for you to open up to your natural ability to self-heal: the self-healing process of your own physical body. This has many stages and aspects to it. Each aspect is not difficult, but each step of the process needs to be explored and experienced, and each step you take is very important. You will find that each step will bring you back toward healing a part of yourself.

As you move into this self-healing process you will begin to open up into a very different relationship with your physical body. You begin to bring your awareness and connection to each individual cell. Your *conscious* awareness to your cells is essential to all physical self-healing.

As you bring your conscious awareness to your cells, the cells begin to open up to a different energetic connection to you and a different relationship to you. They begin to flow with a new rhythm and a new life force—almost a new heart beat. They actually begin to align to an energetic flow or rhythm that connects them to the higher Self, and a pulse begins to become activated that connects them directly to the Universal heartbeat. This new flow of life force within the cell actually begins to create a healing process within all the cells of the body, so the dense energy connected to illness transforms and the body heals. It allows the organs of the body to regenerate with new life force.

The membrane on the outside lining of the cell is opened up energetically and expanded. The cell's membrane is then able to act as a receiver for this light connection. The spaces between the cells can then expand with this new light, and there is fluidity within and around the cell.

Your body's cells are incredibly regenerative, and respond quickly to your *conscious* connection to them. As you consciously open up to the cells, they can begin this journey of their physically healing—this journey of transformation. Remember: This is your body; these are your cells. It's important for you to consciously claim ownership of the cells of your body, so you can communicate with them. Acknowledging your cells is the first step of communication. Through this interaction you are acknowledging your Self on a new level. *You are your cells*, and as each cell begins to awaken in this way you begin to awaken too. You will experience a huge difference in your physical body. Your body is quickly going to feel more alive. There are new levels of light opening up through the cells, which is the beginning of a changing energy.

You are being introduced to a new energetic aspect of the cells of your body, giving you a new awareness of how the cells in your body can relate to you and how you can relate to them. This new understanding will give you important clarity, allowing you to work intimately in an alignment with the cells. You will be given other tools that will enable you to work more deeply and consciously to co-create your physical healing. The cells hold a consciousness, and, as you and the cells begin to work as a team, dramatic healing processes take place.

When you have this intimate relationship with your cells, your whole body will change. Your body will communicate with you in a completely different way. You will know what your body needs in each moment.

As you work with this new dynamic you will find yourself beginning to transform. You will come into an experience of oneness with all living things on this planet. Your healing accelerates as you are able to receive the love that is available to you within this life force. The cells in your body will be able to utilize this love for self-healing and regeneration.

When you move out of separation you create a natural opening to receive an aspect of your abundance that has been always waiting for you. This helps you move into an accelerated physical self-healing process, which is an important step to taking your power back and regaining yourself on a completely new level.

Dis-ease

Pain is the only way your body can communicate with you when there is some type of dis-ease taking place within your body, whether that is created from an unexpressed emotion, or a physical problem that has developed within the cells/organs of your body. The pain says "pay attention to me." Bring your attention to this area of your body.

Generally, our reaction is to move away from pain, take a painkiller, and get rid of the pain as quickly as possible. The more effective action, which will actually take the pain away and create a healing within you, is to step toward yourself, toward your body, and toward the pain. You decide to connect consciously to your physical body and feel what is there inside the pain, because where there is physical pain, there is always unexpressed emotional pain present in the site.

Unexpressed emotion always gets locked into the cells of your body. Each time you cannot cope with the feelings they lock into the cells of the body. There is a density that begins to build up in the cells, so there is an emotional dis-ease that builds up and this turns into physical disease. So when the physical pain begins, the body is saying "Feel me."

Your next step is to bring your consciousness toward the pain and take a breath. The breath needs to be through the mouth, not through the nose. The Conscious Breath more easily opens you up to the feelings. At first the pain may increase; this is good. It's good because it's a sign that you are connected to the site. Bring your consciousness deeper into the pain and take another Conscious Breath. It is helpful to give the pain a color or a form; what does it feel like and look like?

As you move deeper into the pain you may feel some sort of emotion. Some of the process is about opening up to the feelings that need to be expressed, so allow your body to express those feelings so it can move out the emotional pain, and the physical pain can leave.

You may feel as though you need to move your body; this is also good. Don't force the body to move, or contrive movements. The body's movement is automatic. By bringing your consciousness fully into the movement as it happens, you connect to the movement and become part of the experience. The more you are able to be a full part of the experience the more completely the issue can cleanly leave the body. Conscious (mouth) breath will also help you connect into the experience, and help you move out the emotional issue in the cells. It is essential during this process to only work with the Conscious Breath; in and out of the mouth. Be sure that your breath is slow and deep. A fast breath moves you away from experiencing the emotional issue fully, so you want to slow your breath down and bring your consciousness into the site as you breathe.

Sound is another way that blocked energy and the emotional issue can leave the cells of the body. As you take that Conscious Breath, let a small sound come with the out breath. You cannot just create a sound; it's as though a sound moves through you. As you open up to the sound with your consciousness you may have the experience of becoming the sound. When this happens it's as though you move into another state. You begin to experience a deep feeling inside of you as the emotional issue in the cells begins to leave the body. There is a huge release of emotional energy as this happens. The density is gone and then it is possible for healing light to enter your cells. Now, your healing can take place.

You do not have to be aware of the content of the issue. Actually, it helps not to know because then the ego mind cannot begin to interfere with your process. My experience is that, if it is important for you to understand and know what issue is leaving the body, then it is revealed to you during your process.

It's important to understand that all deep issues that hold in the body generally leave in layers. For true healing you need to be able to integrate the different layers of the issue fully within yourself. So be aware that you may be dealing with one layer of an issue, and then another layer of the same issue may surface and you will then deal with another level of emotion from that issue. The journey itself is powerful. Like peeling an onion, there are many layers to come off, so be patient with yourself and open to the energy of your journey of self-healing.

Honor each step that you take and allow the unfolding of your own process. The way for each person to unfold is different, and we all have an individual healing process. You cannot compare your journey to anyone else's, and it's important not to let the ego mind start judging you on your steps. Have a devotion to yourself and a deep appreciation for your self-resurrection.

As you work with yourself in this way you will feel a deep sense of freedom—a sense of lightness as you let go of the layers of emotion that have been holding in your cells. As you work through the layers, know that these issues will not come back. They are gone because you have chosen to meet the feelings, and the issue no longer needs to be held in the body.

I went through my own healing process with Systemic Lupus. I came to the realization that I had an incredible amount of unresolved trauma from my childhood that I had never dealt with, and that trauma was still held in the cells of my body.

When the pain first began in my body I didn't pay attention to it. The emotional dis-ease needed to be expressed, but I was unable to understand this at the time. Then the physical disease took hold of me. I wanted someone to fix me and take away the pain. It did not occur to me to take any responsibility or part in my physical healing. When I did finally wake up and realize that I needed to work with my internal emotions, and realized that I needed to take back the responsibility for my own healing, that is the moment I began to take my power back. That's when my true healing process began.

These thoughts about the healing process were not mine; they were inspired thoughts given to me by an aspect of my light Self. At that time when I was so ill, I was closed off to anything creative. I didn't have an original thought in my head. The one thing I did recognize was the truth of what these inspired thoughts held for me. I was able to recognize the truth, and for that I am forever grateful to myself. I really didn't understand this process, but I knew I had to trust in what was being shown to me. I had some spiritual force pushing me forward toward myself—a part of myself that had been lost to me for so long. Through this connection to Spirit I was given insights and understandings about myself, and my process. It did not feel as though these thoughts were really coming from me; in retrospect I know they came from an aspect of my light Self, and many spiritual helpers.

It took all of my courage to begin to meet some of the deep emotional issues from my past. I began to navigate my way through some of the old wounds that I carried. The process was excruciatingly painful, but there was also incredible relief as I unraveled myself, and felt a new level of me emerging into life.

I can say now that it was the best thing to ever happen to me. It turned me around in my life, and brought me from a place of death into living. I have continued to move more and more into being alive since that time of my illness. Each day I commit to moving more, and more, into life.

You do not need to bring yourself to the edge as I did—unless of course you do. You may need that experience for yourself like I did.

The most important aspects of this beginning process are the attention that you give to the cells of your body and the awakening of a new relationship between you and your cells. Your cells hold the key to your healing, so it is essential to recognize the truth that you are your cells, and build a relationship of oneness with them. This happens automatically with this process, a reunion with your cells, as you begin to connect consciously.

Working With the Cells

Your body is made up of billions of cells. How are you going to work with all these cells? This is actual an easy process. Let's talk about how you can begin to have a direct experience of connecting to your cells and beginning your healing process.

Step 1

Open up your consciousness and acknowledge the existence of all the cells in your body. As you do so, your energy automatically begins to flow to all the cells. You do not have to struggle with this; just let go and allow your energy to naturally flow to each cell. Remember: The universal law is that when you bring your attention/consciousness to something, energy automatically goes to where you place your attention. So, as you bring your consciousness to the cells they begin to feel the conscious connection from you, they begin to open and respond, they begin to change! You begin to change!

Step 2

While you are consciously connecting in this way to the cells you need to simply take a breath, in through the mouth, and then out through the mouth, letting the outward breath go without controlling it. Simply let it go. When you do this, the breath will automatically go to every cell in this physical body of yours. The Pleiadians call it the "Sweeping Breath" because it automatically sweeps through every cell of your body, and in that moment every cell begins to respond to this conscious connection by you. It is the same as the Conscious Breath.

Remember that this Conscious Breath says two things: "Yes, I'm willing to let go of what is holding in my cells," and "Yes, I'm willing to receive my light and my healing through my cells."

So, what is actually happening from this sweeping, Conscious Breath is a letting go in all of the cells in your body. The cells begin letting go of the stress, struggle, and tiredness that has built up in the cells over this lifetime and other lifetimes. As this dense energy leaves the cells it makes it possible for a new level of your light to come into the cells. The cell's membrane is able to transform its energy opening up the cell to receive healing light. This activates the energy of the self-healer and the cells begin to regenerate.

Each cell has a central heart, so, as you open to the cell, the heartbeat or pulse begins to awaken. It's like feeding the smallest flicker of a light, and that light expands into a flame. Your cell needs to be that flame in order for healing to take place. Your cells need love, and the light of the Self brings that love to every cell, awakening each one and activating the individual consciousness of each one. A new life force enters the cell. As the cells begin to flourish, the outer membranes of the cells transform. They become more radiant, and there will be a soft purple light found in the membrane itself, which you may even sense or see.

The cell receives nutrition through this outer membrane, and as the membrane transforms it is able to take in greater nutrition. The space between the cells will expand, allowing each cell to hold a more individual aspect of the Self. The spaces between the cells hold the connection to the other dimensional aspects of you, the healing aspects of Self. So as the spaces open up, the self-healing principle is naturally activated within you.

Sometimes you will experience physical pain as the dense areas open up and leave the body. To accelerate the dense areas leaving, simply bring your attention to where the pain is in the physical body and use the Conscious Breath. Remember that it is useful to give the area where you feel the pain, a color and/or a form. Then bring your consciousness to the form or to the color, and breathe directly into it. The pain may become more intense in that moment, which is the issue leaving the body.

This journey with the cells is about you being willing to receive yourself in a whole different way—being willing to open to this aspect of your body. It is powerful, empowering, and very beautiful. It is an incredible event to witness, this physical birthing of your Self; you taking back your power to self-heal.

Healing Specific Areas of Your Body

Let's look at how you can work with healing specific areas or problems that exist in your own body. You can heal an existing problem in your body by beginning to open up to this new relationship with your cells. Once the relationship is established you can then begin to work on the specific site of your body, in partnership with the cells. It does not matter where in the body your problem exists; it can be a small problem or an acute problem. It can be in an organ, muscles, bone, or a body system. All healing processes are met in the same way, first working with establishing a new relationship with your cells, and then working with the specific area in your body.

If the problem is in a specific area you need to bring your consciousness into the area. This area will have certain denseness to it. Your focus and intention need only be to feel what is in the cells. Begin to bring your consciousness into the space, let go, and bring your Conscious Breath inside the space. As you do this, explore this area with your mind and ask yourself what color is here, and what does this area feel like: Is it fluid, soft, hard, hot, or cold? Once you have a sense of what it feels like, begin to bring your conscious into this area and use the Conscious Breath. Keep working within the site step by step, moment by moment. Don't rush; just be committed to your process with your body. You can do it slowly a piece at a time, or move more quickly. It depends on the type of issue you are dealing with within your body.

The bigger the physical problem taking place in your body, the larger the emotional issue that is holding there. Be committed to opening up to the whole area of the emotional issue, and keep feeling the dense area and the changes that take place within the site as you let go. As the area begins to open up you will feel as though a burden has been lifted off your shoulders and you will have a new sense of freedom. Continue the process until the site has completely transformed and your healing is completed.

In my own healing experience, I had such a wonderful sense of achievement as I opened up to into this process and was able to open up to my body in a new way. I began to have a completely different connection to and relationship with my physical body. There was an intimacy between my body and me; I could feel what it needed in the terms of nutrition, exercise, sleep, and leisure.

I also noticed that I had a different sense of my connection to nature and how my body received from the natural forces: how my body actually received energy and nutrition from nature. It was wonderful feeling connected into my body for the first time in my life.

I became aware that my thoughts about myself were sent to my body, and were taken in by my cells. I needed to begin to love this physical form of mine, to continue to open to a self-loving principle with my cells. As I did so my healing accelerated. So be aware of the messages you send to your physical body and to examine how you feel about your body. It has a direct impact on your cells.

The most important thing in this journey of self-healing is to know that it is a step-by-step process of change. You do not have to do it perfectly. Set your intention and take one step at a time. And you do not have to do it alone. You have the help and support of the Spiritual realms and the Pleiadians; just open up and ask for the help.

◇◇◇◇◇◇◇◇◇◇◇◇◇

The 11th audio track (*www.christinedayonline.com/piol/*) was created so that you can connect back to a direct communication with your cells, and begin a new relationship with them and with your whole body. The work you will do here with these audio files will be a catalyst for you to return to your self-healing of your physical body. We hold you in great love as you move into this transformation of the cells and healing in your physical body. Work with these audio files as many times as necessary until the transformation and the healing of yourself is complete.

With much love—

Chapter 12
Cocoon Work

You are now ready to begin your work with the Cocoon. The Cocoon is an energetic form that you are going to create for yourself; it is multidimensional and will be birthed uniquely for you. Energies are going to be held open for you by the Pleiadians that will allow you to create this energetic form to help you grow and rejuvenate within your physical, spiritual, and emotional bodies. The best way to describe this Cocoon is to liken it to returning to the womb. It allows you to grow in energetic ways, and yet it takes you into a deep rest state. This rest state is different from anything you can access on this earth plane; of course it is this multidimensional form that will hold you as you move through a deep metamorphosis process within your body. It allows you to de-stress your nervous system, and this affects all the cells in your body.

The Cocoon energy has an amazing, safe, and nurturing environment that activates a self-regeneration process within the physical, emotional, and spiritual levels. The formation of your Cocoon enables you to activate a process of cellular regeneration within your system and for a deep healing to take place within your cells. It allows you to receive new levels of your divine light into the cells and for you to align to the multidimensional aspects of the Self. It will also be able to assist you with the integration of your energies as you birth yourself in your awakening of the Self.

When you are in the Cocoon there is an energetic that allows the cells to be in a deep resting place. As you rest in the Cocoon the stress in the cells flows out, and the energy of your body is restored to a new, balanced level so that you can realign to the natural energies of the Self.

The energy that is created in the Cocoon is at a different dimensional level than you have experienced so far in this work. When I say different I mean that the energy that is present in the Cocoon opens an energetic especially for your rejuvenation, and your experience will be deep and may be unfamiliar to your previous experiences up to this point. There is such a unique aspect to the energy that forms for you here in your Cocoon; it is a unique birthing and integrating energy. Your system needs this, especially with the awakening energies you have taken in from the journeys in the Stargate and Formation. It's especially helpful if you are in the process of physical and emotional self-healing. It will accelerate your healing process because of the deep rest state that it provides.

Your Cocoon is here to assist you to more fully integrate the transformations that are taking place within you, so that your alignments to your Self can be integrated more easily, and you can move into a natural flow with your Self on many more levels.

The energy of the Cocoon holds you constantly within this energetic resting place, and once it is activated it will assist you in your ongoing transformation. The Cocoon is another tool for you, bringing deeper integrations with these new awakening states. But more important, the Cocoon holds you on an ongoing daily basis, surrounding you energetically as you move through your world and holding you in a deep rest space.

The Cocoon is also a healing place for your inner kids to be because they feel held within this space. There is a sense of safety for them so they can truly rest. For those of us who have had a traumatic childhood, the Cocoon is a safe harbor, so those inner kids who are so afraid can let go of some of their fear and begin to get the rest they so completely need. Healing for them can begin, so some of their deeper wounds have a chance to heal, creating a resurrection process for them within this space.

There are many advantages to allowing your inner child to help you in building your Cocoon. An inner child brings an energy to the Cocoon that you can utilize—an energy that you don't necessarily have access to. These inner kids have an essence of innocence and sweetness in their hearts; this energy is woven into your Cocoon. That's why it is an advantage to you, and very helpful to allow your inner child, or children, to be a part of the experience of building your Cocoon. Their energies are pure and powerful as they bring a creativity to the project of building your Cocoon, and most importantly they bring the energy of joy.

Building your Cocoon can be a joint effort and a wonderful way to connect to your child. It is sometimes difficult in our busy lives to find time to build a relationship with the inner child, and it is so easy to forget our child aspects. In the Cocoon, you and your child share the experience, and it can heal some of your separation issues. This connection to the child in your life is very important and can bring you many gifts. You need this connection to your inner child to be complete within yourself, and your child has some important aspects to bring that you need for your own healing.

There are many individual journeys for you to experience within the Cocoon. Each time the Cocoon will expand on some level and you will find a deeper experience and connection to it. In each journey you will experience a birth within yourself. The actual building process of your Cocoon can be a deep and peaceful experience; just let yourself go into the full creative, energetic process and allow an unlimited flow to take you as you create.

Be aware that you may see, sense, or feel the Cocoon. It does not matter how you personally experience it. It can vary in size: It can be huge, or sometimes it is very small. This is your personal energetic space that will expand in all sorts of ways. It is multidimensional in form, and unlimited energetically. Because it is a fourth-, fifth-, and sixth-dimensional structure you need to remember any experience is possible here. The ego mind will not understand or be able to follow the logic of this space and the experiences you have here. So you need to truly let go and allow yourself to move with the adventure of many experiences as you unfold with your Cocoon. You are being asked to let go and not to let the ego mind begin assessing what you are doing, or how you are doing it. Let go and allow yourself to enjoy this space freely. Use your breath as you build your Cocoon. Bring your consciousness to parts of the Cocoon as it begins to form and breathe as you build the structure; it's like breathing a life force into your Cocoon.

Connecting Into the Body

You need to be connected into your physical body as you build your Cocoon, to be more connected to the experiences taking place within the Cocoon, and to form a deeper relationship with the Cocoon and with the energy that is within the Cocoon. Bring your hands to your chest area, feel your hands meeting at your chest, and do your Conscious Breathing.

Keep focusing into your body while you are in the Cocoon, energetically connected to your heart, so you will be able to utilize and connect to the Cocoon's energy. Breathe and let go, allowing yourself to rest within your Cocoon space.

During your work within the Cocoon it is important that you do not try to visualize things, or try to make things happen with the mind. This will stop your true experience. It will move you away from what is actually happening. The ego mind is unable to work within the energetic space of the Cocoon. It cannot function here, so when you try to visualize an experience you move out of the energy of the Cocoon. You don't want the mind to control this process. When an experience just comes to you naturally, bring your attention to it and take a breath. The energy of the experience will expand. You can trust each step of your experiences here; you can trust your breath and just allow the Cocoon to build and form in each moment.

It's important to be in each moment and to use the Conscious Breath with each experience. But you are going to be asked to let go, and allow yourself to fully receive during this Cocoon process and to be willing to allow yourself to receive on many new levels. Everything within the Cocoon space is for you to utilize for yourself; it's a true space just for you to receive, and, because you are dealing with many different dimensional spaces, there are unlimited possibilities within the Cocoon for you to receive. Many types of experiences can take place for you here. It does not need to make sense on a third-dimensional level, remember that you have moved out of this third-dimensional space.

How to Activate and Build Your Cocoon

You are going to need a candle for this process. The candle can be any color and it needs to be at least 6 inches in height. You do not want a scented candle, because when you are in other dimensional spaces your senses are heightened and the smell will possibly interfere with some of your experiences. Always use the same candle for the Cocoon, and keep this candle just for your Cocoon work.

The lighting of your candle is significant. It is symbolic of opening up the energy of your Cocoon, with the pure light of the flame and the fluidity of the flame. These aspects of the flame reflect some of the energies of your Cocoon so as you light the candle, each time, your Cocoon will automatically respond. The light of the candle expands through the Cocoon, building it in size and energy, and the energy that anchors you in the Cocoon begins to birth through the cells of your body, especially the heart. The energy of the candle helps to activate an alignment process through your cells of the heart, so that the heart opens and flows with the Cocoon. The candle transmits a pure energy. The light of the flame holds fluidity, and purity, and these energies play their part in the building of the Cocoon.

Step 1

Sit down on the floor with the candle in front of you. Be sure you have plenty of room around you, so that your arms can go fully out to the sides without touching anything else, or anybody else. Before lighting your candle take a few breaths and open up to an intention for yourself. Be consciously open to receiving what it is that your need for yourself.

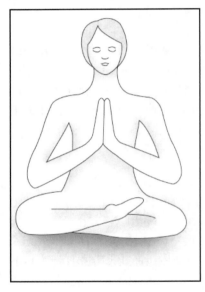

Diagram H

Light the candle.

Begin with the palms of the hands together at the heart. (See Diagram H.) Bring your full attention to the hands, and take a sweeping breath through the cells of your body. Then bring your full attention/consciousness back to your hands. Feel energy begin to form between your hands as you bring your consciousness to them. There will be energy that begins to build here; it will build between your hands and through the center of yourself. As you bring your consciousness to this building energy it will begin to expand. Remember: Your breath will open the energy even more as you bring your consciousness to this place.

Gradually you will begin to experience a focused core of light beginning to form within you, within your center, and between the hands.

To expand this core, bring your focus/attention to where the hands meet and breathe. As you do this you will become aware of a deeper line of energy anchoring even more completely through you. This is the beginning of the core. Every time you bring your energy there, the core will expand in some way. You may see or sense this.

Be sure you are relaxed. There is no need to rush; you can take your time. This is your journey—your moment. Take the time just to be with yourself and with your experience.

When you are ready, bring your attention to the flame of the candle; watch the flame and breathe. The energy of the flame will begin to open up into you. Be with the purity of the flame, and the fluidity of the flame. Open consciously to the light coming from the flame, and open up to receive this light. You will experience this energy from the flame coming into your core and also opening up into the building energy in between your hands.

Now bring your focus to where the palms of the hands are at your heart, and breathe. The core will expand again. You may feel the light from the candle feeding into your core, building and expanding your core outward.

You need to repeat this entire process of building the energy of your core and connecting to the flame as many times as you need to. There will come a point where the energy that is building between the hands needs to move. As you feel this buildup of energetic pressure you will begin to move your hands outward to each side, as far out as your arms can stretch. (See Diagram I.)

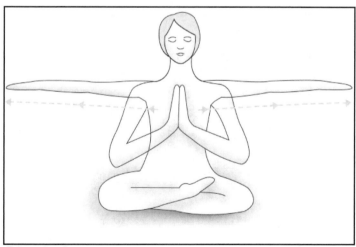

Diagram I

Step 2

Begin to move your hands slowly apart, moving them out sideways. As you do this the buildup of light energy from your hands and your core begins to flow out with your movement. This is where your Cocoon begins to birth itself. This light energy will expand in its own way, as it creates the beginning form of your energetic Cocoon. It will have a life of its own—its own unique pattern and form. Just let the form expand and create itself. Witness this unfolding and breathe. Let go and allow. This is the beginning stage of your Cocoon birthing from the light from the core.

Step 3

Now bring your hands from the sides slowly upward to above your head. Your palms come upward above your head until the palms meet together. (See Diagram J.) As you do this you will experience the light energy from the core begin to open up on another energetic level, creating the sides and top of your Cocoon. When you do this movement, the light will begin to expand up and out, opening the energy of your Cocoon even more completely, which is the beginning of the full form of your Cocoon. Bring your consciousness to your hands above your head, and feel the energy, breathe, and let the energy expand.

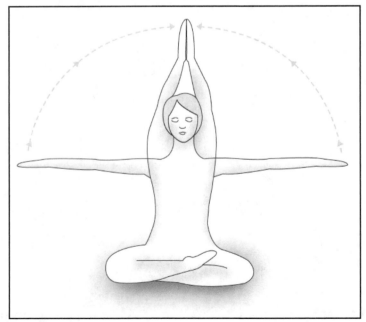

Diagram J

Step 4

As you connect to the energy in your hands as they are held above your head, open up to the sense of the energy around you, and just be with the feeling here. When you sense it is time, bring your hands straight down, as though you are moving down through the core of yourself and back to the central heart position. (See Diagram K.)

Feel the energy when you do this. As you move your hands down through the core, there will be a deeper alignment taking place within you to the Cocoon, and as you bring your consciousness to your central core there is an even more expanded light birthing through your core, expanding and strengthening itself, and flowing down through your center.

As you bring your consciousness back to your connected palms, feel how the core expands through the center of the body creating an expansion or change within the Cocoon itself. The Cocoon will expand out, growing in depth and transforming from the center outward. The light of your core will become more radiant as it is pulsing outward, filling in the sides of your Cocoon and into the base of your

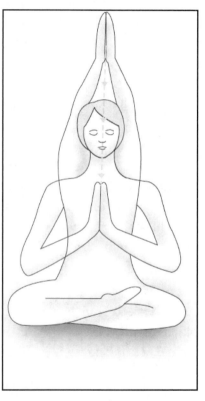

Diagram K

Cocoon. This may be a very strong visual or a sensory experience, or it can be subtle; it does not matter with regard to the effectiveness of building your Cocoon. Allow it to have a life of its own and to unfold as it needs to. If your experience is subtle, bring your consciousness to the subtlety and breath, and open up to these subtle energies.

◇◇◇◇◇◇◇◇◇◇◇◇◇

It's important as you complete your first cycle of this process that you rest in the energy of the form in the Cocoon that has already birthed. Rest at your heart, feeling the connection to the core, opening to the light of the candle, and opening to the beginning form of your Cocoon. It's important also to connect deeply to the core of your Cocoon as you rest. When you feel ready to continue, repeat the process and let go, allowing your Cocoon to birth itself on another level. Know that your Cocoon has a life of its own. You cannot control how it forms; it brings to you exactly what you need for your rest and rejuvenation.

Each time you repeat a cycle of this movement from the heart back to the heart, your Cocoon will expand on many levels, and, as it does, you also will expand and change. As it develops and expands, you need to bring the light of the flame of the candle into the Cocoon even more completely. The flame plays a big part in the transformation of the Cocoon, and, each time you open to the flame, another aspect of the fluidity of the flame's energy weaves itself into the Cocoon. This weaving transforms the energy of your Cocoon, building and expanding its light form. Know that this light form is part of the multidimensional layers that will create your healing Cocoon.

Only work with the light of the flame when you feel drawn to the flame; you don't have to do it every time. Know that when your hands come back to your heart you can rest; the heart position is your resting place. Just be in your core until you feel it is time to build more of your Cocoon space. It is up to you when you do more building of the Cocoon.

You will have a feeling of completeness at the end of each Cocoon journey. That is when you will stop building the Cocoon, knowing it is not finished yet but compete for now. The energies in the Cocoon have expanded enough for your next step. Don't overwork yourself trying to build your Cocoon all at one time. When you feel your Cocoon is complete for now, it's time to rest within your Cocoon. Lie down or sit in this space, letting yourself deeply rest, letting go, and allowing all levels of yourself to take in the energies that are within your Cocoon.

Remember to use your breath through your cells as you rest in this multidimensional space. The stress is able to leave the cells, and the cells' regeneration can take place. There is a deep metamorphosis that will begin to take place within your energetic field and within the cells of your body. Let go and allow this deep rest as you are held within the Cocoon space. Note: Always rest in the Cocoon after it is completed at the end of each journey.

You can return to building your Cocoon on an ongoing basis. Each time it will transform on another level. It is a healing tool for you and, most important, a deep resting place for you that creates a deep rejuvenating process for your cells.

◇◇◇◇◇◇◇◇◇◇◇◇

Now it is time to listen to the channeled audio tracks.

This 12th audio track (*www.christinedayonline.com/piol/*) has been energetically designed by the Pleiadians to assist you in your alignment to your unique Cocoon.

Open the 12th audio track found online. Let go and allow your own unique process to unfold within the Cocoon.

Remember: You need to invite your inner child to be with you on this journey. Inner children bring a lot of creativity to your Cocoon, as well as an essence of innocence.

You are being held in love as you allow this regeneration process to take place within all levels of yourself. We witness and celebrate you as you begin your journey in the building of your Cocoon!

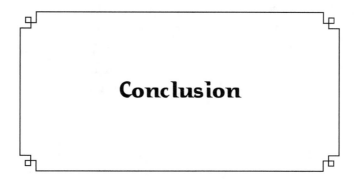

Conclusion

Blessing to All Who Have Read This Book and Taken Their Places Within the Universal Consciousness Through Each Initiation

At this time there is a huge wave of light frequencies energy going outward across your planet. The Pleiadians are expanding the work out to all of you, and you are playing your role. They have told me that this energy would go through a tremendous expansion beginning the year 2009, the year this "Self Healing Prophecy" was activated on our planet. This energy is building momentum, like a huge wave it moves out, rippling throughout the world. Each one of you is participating in this energy building; each of you has a unique part to play as you go through your initiations with this book. You are anchoring your light into the cells of your body, automatically transmitting your light energy onto the planet, taking your place. I honor you for doing this.

It feels like I am being lined up energetically on a new level to work in a completely new way in the world, with the Frequencies work and with holding large transmitting energies for large groups of people. I share this with you because you are a part of that: your energy. Your unique divine aspect is a part of the energetic wave that is supporting our planet now. The energy we are working with here in this book is a strong and profound energy. It feels like a new level of love becoming accessible to mankind and a new wave of light work being anchored on the planet.

There are absolutely no accidents. Each one of you has come to take your place by opening up to the initiating energies of this book, and each one of you is being held and honored for opening up to the initiations. You are meant to be here at this time doing this work, and the initiations bring us all together as part of the collective. This is part of the Self Healing Prophecy: the alignment to oneness, so that we begin to directly experience our place in the oneness here on this earth plane. We claim our place and begin to flow together in one consciousness and together we create an amazing light force.

We've all made a pre-agreement to be here at this time. We meet on this energetic level. Yes, we can meet on the physical, but we meet on the energetic level—the energetic planes with our own soul essence and our own light selves.

The Pleiadians want you to understand the significance of you taking your place at this time, because the most important thing is your conscious action, with every action you take in every moment. Your conscious action says "Yes, I have chosen to come here. I have come to take my place. I have come here to birth myself back into wholeness." It is about consciously taking your steps forward at this time, not just drifting through your life—conscious action and conscious thought, saying "Yes, I am here. I claim my place here. I take my place. I receive myself, and my initiation, now. I claim every cell in this body. I claim my light and allow every cell to anchor my light. I am alive."

The time for us to act on this is now. Being alive is opening up and allowing that light connection to the Self into the cells, acknowledging every cell in your body and consciously saying *yes* with every breath into every cell. It is not letting the fear of the ego stop you in any way, but living through your heart and being in the strength of your sacred heart connection.

As you live this conscious action of receiving your own life force and anchoring it through the cells of your body, you align with your pure life force and flow of your light.

I go back to my experience of dying in Banneux, trying to get back into my body when my body was cold. My physical body had died. I can still go back into that terrible feeling—the shock of that moment. Not only shock—despair. I still had a lot to do here on this earth plane. My life was over, and my body was gone. Mary came to me in that moment and said you have completed everything you said you were going to do here in your lifetime. So it was time for me to leave. I said to her at the time, "No, this is not right; I have too much to do here and I have to go back." She told me I had to open up to a whole new commitment to this lifetime and create a new blueprint. I've come to realize it was at that time that I was really able to understand the importance for me to be here, to live this life, and to bring another level of myself here. I made another commitment, actually another commitment to myself at that time, and that was to live more and to be even more alive. And I was able to come back into my body. Everything inside of me started to light up. A pure light moved right through my cells and my body came back to life.

This experience took me a whole year to fully integrate. I stayed away from the experience for a long time. I didn't truly meet the experience; I just went on living and I needed to integrate. I didn't go to the experience to explore the depth of it because it was just too much for me to digest, but I did have an awareness that it was important for me to return to it when I was able to. When I did finally align back to that moment I relived those deep emotions of needing to live and the importance of being here on the planet now. I needed the experience to truly know how important it is to be on this earth plane now, and I am grateful that I had the opportunity and was given the grace to return here to continue my life. I am much more anchored and even more committed to living here in a new conscious way and appreciation for being alive.

Your consciously saying *yes* to being here is essential. Being caught up in the third-dimensional illusion, in the struggle, in the fear, in the tiredness, in the "It's so hard, I just want to be happy"—all the third-dimensional ego talk. The illusion prevents you from aligning to you. Just begin to refuse these messages from the ego. Remember: You choose love or fear each moment. Open up to love and you open up to the connection to your heart; open up to fear and you open your connection to the ego mind.

It is a big decision to be here as human beings living on this earth plane at this time. It's a huge decision and a great privilege to be allowed to be here at this time. It's important to actually remember you chose to be here: Every day you choose to be here.

You are being asked now to move in a different way and to be conscious of being here. Yes, there are third-dimensional pieces we have to move through, but we have magnificence in ourselves! We can live through our hearts, and allow more of ourselves to be here in a new way—willing to walk through the world *consciously*, consciously aligning to our magnificence.

It's time to move away from the agony of the third dimension. The fact is, we are playing out a role here, but we can move into a magnificent state of flowing and allowing the light of ourselves to take us through our lives. We can stop being so afraid. Each one of you has come to this book to birth yourself in a new way. You've answered your destiny call. This call is not a third-dimensional call. It is the call of Spirit, the truth, the alignment of your light that has brought you to this moment. It's your true Spirit, your true Self, that is birthing through you, and the whole Universe is witnessing you in this birth.

I hold the space for you to birth consciously—to breathe and let the feelings come.

The feelings can be there, but don't let the fear grab you and tie you down. Recognize the illusion, breathe, connect into your heart, and keep stepping forward to open to the love and the connection to Self. This is *your* place that you are taking in the world. You make a difference, your point of light being consciously active in the world. Consciously open to this truth, claim this truth about yourself, and anchor and activate this on an energetic level within the universe, on this planet. Then your energy can be utilized as it was always meant to be. Don't minimize your place here. Don't minimize your magnificence and the anchoring of your energy. There is not one of us that is less than the other. We each hold an equal energetic place and when we are in that space we can hold an aspect of an energetic flow that makes a difference.

Your ego mind cannot make a difference to your magnificence. It cannot make a dent in it because you are whole and complete in your energy. The difference is whether you close off from yourself or not. Your brilliance never goes away; it never stops being in its complete form.

The questions are how willing you are to completely embrace yourself in this form of light, and how willing you are to embrace and utilize the incredible form of light in your day to day living. Are you willing to utilize the energetic support that is here for you from the universe, the spiritual forces, the Pleiadian energies, and all the energies, supporting us to be masters of ourselves on a new level, in a realignment to the Self?

You don't have to be afraid when you turn back to the Self. You understand that this journey here on this earth plane is a return back to the Self, aligning to the light of the Self and to your divine uniqueness. No else holds your energy but you. All you have to do is begin activating your place through a conscious desire.

Consciously claim your place and claim your pre-agreement to be here on this earth plane today. Acknowledge the place you are taking and the commitment. Activate your claim with the words *I am.* You are claiming your Self right now. And remember the words *Thy Will Be Done.* You are speaking to the light aspect of yourself, saying "I will follow thy will, the will of the light of the Self." You are here to claim your natural birth right of Self.

So be it.

I hold the space and the platform for each one of you to birth yourself. I honor each one of you for showing up for your pre-agreement. Whether you are aware of what brought you here or not, you are here. You have navigated yourself here. You are not alone in this glorious journey; you are being held in love each step. Remember that we are here.

Keep moving forward, consciously, toward your freedom.

With love and blessings,

Christine

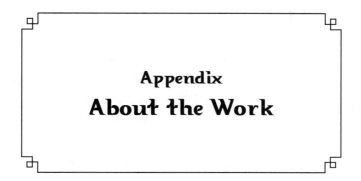

Appendix
About the Work

It feels important that I talk about, and describe to you, the two bodies of work that were channeled to me so long ago and that are currently being offered in many areas of the world today.

Amanae was the first channeled work that I anchored into the world. Amanae is a hands-on, multi-dimensional bodywork process that opens up the emotionally held blocks in the body. Amanae opens up a direct access for you to connect to your emotions that are held in your physical body. As you consciously *feel* this emotion, it can leave your body, and healing can take place. This moves the body into healing on many different levels, within the physical and emotional bodies. And there is a deep spiritual transformation that takes place as the emotion moves out, and the light of the Self anchors into your cells.

Frequencies of Brilliance was channeled through me, and birthed at the exact same moment as Amanae. At the time these two bodies of work were anchored through me, I was told humans were not ready for this second body of work, so it was not to be transmitted on to the earth plane at that time. Thirteen years later, in 1999, I was told to begin teaching and initiating people in this work, and it was to be called Frequencies of Brilliance. I have been initiating practitioners and teachers in this work ever since, and it has been my main work on the earth plane since that time.

What Is This Work?

Frequencies of Brilliance is fourth/fifth- and sixth-dimensional work, and it creates a powerful, multidimensional healing energy that is above and far beyond what this third-dimension earth plane can provide. Because this energy is from the higher dimensional levels it opens up and allows for advanced physical and emotional healing to take place with each person. An important role of this work is to also create accelerated spiritual awakenings through light initiations. These powerful initiations are designed to work uniquely with each person for whatever level they are at in the moment, bringing deep personal direct experiences from the Spiritual realms and the Pleiadians. This work aligns you to new aspects of your light Self and anchors this light into the cells of your body for your awakening.

The Pleiadians have crafted a series of light initiations designed to awaken the human being to be aligned to the Spiritual Self. They use the sacred geometrical forms for some of the initiations, and work within the Stargate spaces with you for other higher-level initiations.

Many of the healings associated with the Frequency of Brilliance have been called miraculous, yet in truth they are simply healings that are made possible when associated with the fourth-, fifth-, and sixth-dimensional spaces. These energies connect to the higher levels of Self of the person receiving the work, allowing for deep healing to take place. This is cutting-edge healing work that can accelerate healing processes on a physical and emotional level, and take that person on the Spiritual path to an accelerated awakening.

The Pleiadians are truly amazing in how they channeled through to me these different processes that are so dynamic and powerful. And even more remarkable is that all these processes bypass the ego mind, which is incredibly helpful to us as human beings.

How to Learn About the Work

The Stage I work of Frequencies of Brilliance is a 13- to 14-day training and initiation process. These initiations are based on aligning to higher levels of the aspects of the Self through a series of re-alignments with the use of sacred geometrical forms, which activate and open other dimensional spaces, and then working within these spaces with the help of the Pleiadian and Spiritual forces. The Pleiadians and the Spiritual energies assist in the initiations throughout the training and you begin to develop your own personal relationship with the Pleiadians, and deepen your connection and conscious awareness to the spiritual realms. As you do this you expand with each new alignment to yourself. This Stage 1 process prepares you to become a practitioner of Frequencies of Brilliance. This series of initiations is extremely powerful and highly transformational. Although many people take this training to become a practitioner of the work, others take the training just for the initiations themselves.

I continue to channel new levels of the work, and there are now 12 stages of this work available. Having worked extensively with groups of people during the last 15 years, I have seen the deep changes that take place within each person with the help of these initiation processes. This work has evolved and expanded, as I have been able to expand within myself.

As well as initiating students and teachers in the Frequency of Brilliance processes, I am working with larger groups of people with what are called Transmissions and Pleiadian Seminars.

What Are Transmissions?

Transmissions are energetic sessions channeled by the Pleiadians. They are held in different venues throughout the world and are open to the general public. They usual last one and a half hours. The Transmissions begins with a channeled dialogue from the Pleiadians, so each Transmission tends to work with a theme, and each Transmission is completely different from the other. These Transmissions create healing and energetic transformations, initiating you into a higher level of your light. They are highly transformational and allow you to take another step toward your Self. They work by transmitting healing light out to large groups of people, so everyone within the area receives these energies of light. These transmissions of light open up initiations for you—initiations of the Self through your cells. This can create healing through the physical body and the emotional body, and create new levels of spiritual awakening for each individual.

What Are Pleiadian Seminars?

The newest work that the Pleiadians are opening up for us here is a three-day Pleiadian seminar, an initiation open to the general public. These events have been opened up at this time to work with us to receive more levels of the Self Healing Prophecy. It is a powerful initiation process with the Pleiadians, working within different dimensional spaces, learning how to navigate within these different dimensional spaces, and working within the Stargate chamber with the help of the Pleiadians. This event brings you in direct contact with the Pleiadians, forming a personal relationship with them during the three days and then continuing to work with them in your life. You will be working within fourth/fifth- and sixth-dimensional spaces. I will be channeling the Pleiadian material and energies. There will be information and channeled dialogue throughout this event. There will be opportunities for you to ask questions directly to the Pleiadians during this time.

It is very powerful to come together in groups to experience the work. As larger numbers of people are opened up, there is an accelerated awakening that takes place for each person.

There will be a crystal vortex activated for you to experience and work with, which allows the Pleiadians to work and align with you more completely. It will also allow you to align more easily with the different dimensional spaces that will open. One of my roles is to dial the dimensional spaces within the vortex for you to initiate into and begin to navigate yourself.

Any energies from the spiritual realms are able to come and assist in these events because of the fine energies that are set up for the initiations. It allows the Angels, Light Beings. and Masters to be able to come into the workspace to assist you in your transformations.

Know that there is a place being held for each one of you who choose to come to this event for your next step. I look forward to all of you called to be part of this experience.

For more information about the work, practitioners in your area, the dates of these events, and other inquiries see my Website (*www. frequenciesofbrilliance.com*).

◇◇◇◇◇◇◇◇◇◇◇◇◇

Available to You

Set of 12 CDs

These are expanded energies for each of the 12 Pleiadian chapters in this book. They are designed to take you deeper into your initiation process. It is important that you first work with the accompanying audio files found at *www.christinedayonline.com/piol/* before starting this advanced series. They can be ordered on my Website (*www. frequenciesofbrilliance.com*).

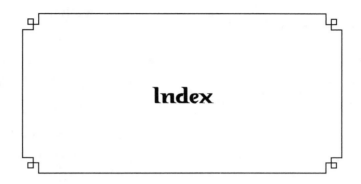

Index

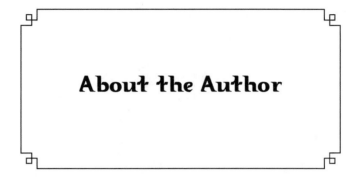

About the Author

C hristine Day currently lives in Minneapolis, Minnesota. She travels the world teaching Frequencies of Brilliance, doing live energetic transmissions from the Pleadians throughout the world, and conducting a three-day "Pleiadian Seminar" open to the general public in the Minneapolis/St. Paul area. She also has a worldwide Webcasting show that is broadcast every second month out of Las Vegas, Nevada. See her Website for more information (*www. frequenciesofbrilliance.com*).

CPSIA information can be obtained
at www.ICGtesting.com
Printed in the USA
FFOW01n0041150815
15884FF